Jackie Bryan   07764·889353

C000226232

Oral anticoagulation mana
and stroke prevention

Edited by DA Fitzmaurice & ET Murray

Published by Hayward Medical Communications

Published by Hayward Medical Communications, a division of Hayward Group Ltd,
The Pines, Fordham Road, Newmarket CB8 7LG, UK.

Copyright © 2009 Hayward Medical Communications.

All rights reserved. No part of this publication may be reproduced, stored in a retrieval
system or transmitted, in any form or by any means, without the prior permission in
writing of Hayward Medical Communications. The data, opinions and statements
appearing in this book are those of the contributor(s) concerned; they are not
necessarily endorsed by the publisher or the Editors. Accordingly, the publisher and its
respective employees, officers and agents accept no liability for the consequences of
any such inaccurate or misleading data, opinion or statement.

ISBN 0 9542022 01

Printed in Great Britain by Latimer Trend.

Contents

Preface

It is with great pleasure and surprise that I am writing the preface to the third edition of this book. It has proved popular with students on the oral anticoagulation courses we run at the National Centre for Anticoagulation Training (NCAT) in Birmingham, where they take great pleasure in pointing out errors or inaccuracies. As in the previous two editions, we have tried to include a little horizon scanning with sections on patient self-management and also new therapeutic agents. Self-management continues to grow as a means of service delivery, and newer agents are now licensed, if only for limited indications, at the time of writing. There is also increasing interest in the use of antithrombotic agents as thromboprophylaxis to prevent thromboembolism as a consequence of hospital admission. This is currently beyond the scope of the book, but may feature in the fourth edition!

I would like to thank all the contributors and also readers for providing critical feedback. I hope this edition proves as successful and useful as the previous two.

DA Fitzmaurice

Chapter 1

How warfarin works

Dr JA Murray

Dr WA Lester

Learning outcomes

- **The principles of the coagulation cascade and how it is affected by warfarin**
- **An understanding of the pharmaceutical interactions of warfarin**

'Coagulation has been studied for years and years by many investigators; none of them can presume that the problem is yet solved.'
Bordet (1921)

Most patients on oral anticoagulation therapy (predominantly warfarin in the UK) are aware that the treatment 'thins the blood'. Normal haemostasis involves interaction between blood vessels, platelets and coagulation factors, and there is a fine balance between procoagulant and anticoagulant factors. With increasing numbers of patients receiving warfarin therapy, the similar balance between the beneficial effects of preventing thromboembolism and the hazardous effects of excessive thinning of the blood needs to be considered.

Coagulation – classical and revised hypotheses

The traditional model of coagulation was a 'cascade', based on laboratory tests that demonstrate sequential enzymatic conversion of inactive precursors of clotting factors to active forms. The intrinsic and extrinsic pathways lead to the final common pathway; this has been a convenient model for the understanding of clot formation and the use of laboratory investigations to monitor different aspects of coagulation (Figure 1.1, page 2). The activated partial thromboplastin time (APTT) measures the activity of the intrinsic system, while the prothrombin time (PT) measures the activity of the extrinsic system. The modification of the PT to the international normalised ratio (INR) has provided a familiar standardised test for the purpose of monitoring oral anticoagulant therapy.

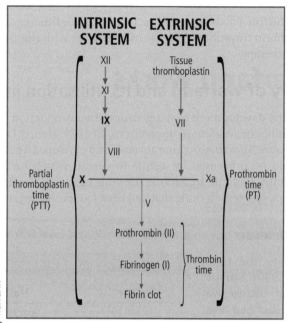

Figure 1.1. A model for understanding clot formation

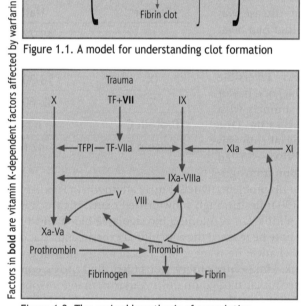

Figure 1.2. The revised hypothesis of coagulation

More recently, it has become clear that this established model does not accurately represent what happens *in vivo*. The revised hypothesis of coagulation (Figure 1.2) differs from the traditional cascade theory in three main respects:
- It integrates all coagulation factors into a single pathway
- It assumes that contact activation is not required *in vivo*
- It assumes that, following the initial generation of factor Xa and thrombin, the haemostatic response must be reinforced or consolidated to progress to completion.

Haemostasis is the fine balance between activators and inhibitors that controls the production of the fibrin thrombus. One way of interfering with this fine balance is by the use of warfarin therapy.

The discovery of warfarin and its utilisation in humans

In common with the development of many drugs, the introduction of warfarin was facilitated by a number of accidental observations. In 1929, Henrik Dam fed chicks a lipid-free diet and found that they became anaemic and developed a tendency to bleed. The bleeding could be prevented by agents in cereals which he nominated the 'Koagulations vitamins' (vitamin K). Around the same time, Karl Paul Link identified a similar haemorrhagic problem in cattle that had been fed spoiled sweet clover.

Sweet clover disease

In the USA, during the Great Depression of the 1930s, a mysterious haemorrhagic disease was observed in cattle that had been fed with spoiled sweet clover hay. It was known that this haemorrhagic disease was reversible either by substituting good hay or by transfusing the animals with blood from healthy cattle. One farmer facing financial ruin was Ed Carlson from Wisconsin. Ed wanted an explanation from agri-

Table 1.1. Vitamin K-dependent factors	
Factor	Half-life
II	48-72 hours
VII	2-6 hours
IX	18-30 hours
X	32-60 hours
Protein C	6 hours
Protein S	42 hours

cultural scientists for his problems. One Saturday afternoon in February 1933, during a blizzard, he drove 190 miles through snow-drifted roads. His truck was laden down with a dead heifer, a milk can containing incoagulable blood and 100 lb of spoiled sweet clover. By the time he reached the agricultural experimental station, the building had closed and, by chance, he reached the biochemistry building where he came across Karl Paul Link. Link's later observations identified a toxic component in the clover as bishydroxycoumarin (dicoumarol). Warfarin, therefore, obtained its name from the Wisconsin Alumni Research Foundation, coupled with the 'arin' from coumarin. The development of Armand Quick's assay for prothrombin in 1936 helped to identify the relationship between vitamin K and warfarin. Further accidental observations were still to come, however. Following its introduction as a very effective rat poison in 1948, it took the accidental poisoning of a US serviceman to demonstrate the possible therapeutic application of warfarin.

Mode of action

Coumarins such as warfarin are vitamin K antagonists that result in reduced biological activity of the vitamin K-dependent factors II, VII, IX and X, as well as proteins C and S

(Table 1.1, page 3). Glutamic acid residues of coagulation proteins require gammacar-boxylation for activation. Warfarin blocks this action, resulting in inactive precursor molecules, termed proteins induced by vitamin K absence. Dietary vitamin K enters the body and is reduced to a hydroquinone form. This reduced form of vitamin K is converted to vitamin K epoxide when it produces the biologically active coagulation

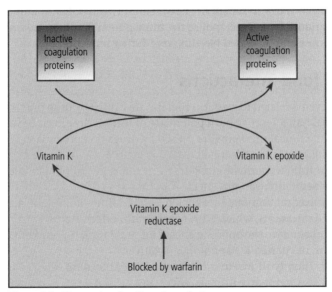

Figure 1.3. The mode of action of warfarin

proteins. In order to regenerate the reduced vitamin K, the enzyme vitamin K epoxide reductase is required. This is the warfarin-sensitive step that is blocked in a competitive fashion by all coumarin-type anticoagulant drugs (Figure 1.3). It is now known that certain genetic variants of vitamin K epoxide reductase (such as VKORC1 Asp36Tyr) can increase a patient's resistance to warfarin, which explains some of the variability in warfarin dose requirements.

The rate by which circulating vitamin K-dependent factors fall and subsequently recover after stopping warfarin is determined by their half-life. A reduction in factor II (prothrombin) is considered particularly important for the antithrombotic effect of coumarins and the long half-life of this clotting factor partly explains the slow onset of anticoagulation over many days from the initiation of drugs like warfarin. In this way, dosing warfarin is rather like navigating a large ocean liner, requiring skill and anticipation. Medical illness in patients taking warfarin should also be considered. For example, if liver impairment occurs (such as in the elderly with congestive cardiac failure), the effect on hepatic metabolism, including further reductions in clotting factors, can increase the INR and the risk of bleeding, and recovery after stopping warfarin can be delayed.

Metabolism of warfarin

Warfarin metabolism primarily takes place in the liver. It exists as a mixture of R- and S-isomers which differ with respect to plasma concentrations, clearance, potency and the cytochrome P450 isoenzymes, which are responsible for metabolism. Sequence variations (genetic polymorphisms) within cytochrome P450 isoenzymes account for some of the variability in warfarin sensitivity between individuals. For example, CYP2C9*2 and *3 allele variants, which metabolise the more potent S-isomer, are associated with lower warfarin dose and increased bleeding risk during induction.

Drug and food interactions

Many adverse events related to warfarin therapy are caused by drug interactions. Drugs and some herbal remedies may both potentiate or inhibit the effects of warfarin. Most of the important clinical problems are caused by drugs that potentiate. There are various types of drug interaction described.

- Displacement from warfarin binding to serum albumin – sulphonamides, phenylbutazone, which enhance warfarin effect.
- Inhibition of liver microsomal breakdown – cimetidine, allopurinol, metronidazole, tricyclic antidepressants, which enhance warfarin effect. Hepatic enzyme inducers such as rifampicin have the opposite effect and cause warfarin resistance.
- Malabsorption of vitamin K – antibiotics, laxatives.
- Aspirin – consistently shown to increase the risk of bleeding when co-administered with warfarin. Rather than a primary effect on warfarin levels or its metabolism, the irreversible inhibition of platelet function by aspirin serves to compromise global clotting potential. The platelet inhibition associated with the commonly used non-steroidal anti-inflammatory drugs (NSAIDs) is more mild and reversible, although they too increase the risk of gastrointestinal haemorrhage, due to their effects on the gut epithelium. Both aspirin and NSAIDs should be used with extreme caution and only when the benefits of co-prescription with warfarin outweigh the risks.

Changes in diet are still poorly understood but can also potentiate the effects of warfarin; for example, cranberry juice can have this effect, probably by impairing warfarin's hepatic metabolism. However, foods containing high quantities of vitamin K, such as green leafy vegetables, reduce the effect of warfarin. Alcohol has a variable and complex interaction, including acute inhibition and chronic enhanced metabolism of warfarin. Some patients will develop a high INR without any change in their diet, alcohol intake or their drug therapy. None of us can presume that the problem is yet resolved, even with our increased appreciation of the pharmacogenetic differences between individuals taking warfarin.

Summary

- Warfarin obtained its name from the Wisconsin Alumni Research Foundation, coupled with the 'arin' from coumarin.
- The prothrombin time (PT) is a laboratory test that measures the activity of the extrinsic system. The modification of the prothrombin time to the international

normalised ratio (INR) is the familiar standardised test for the purpose of monitoring oral anticoagulant therapy.

- Coumarins, such as warfarin, are vitamin K antagonists that result in reduced biological activity of the vitamin K-dependent factors II, VII, IX and X, as well as proteins C and S.
- There is an increasing understanding of the genetic variations that account for some of the differences in warfarin sensitivity between individuals.
- Drugs, herbal remedies, alcohol and food may both potentiate or inhibit the effects of warfarin by different mechanisms.

Further reading
Ansell J, Hirsh J, Hylek E *et al*. Pharmacology and management of the vitamin K antagonists: American College of Chest Physicians Evidence-Based Clinical Practice Guidelines (8th Edition). *Chest* 2008; **133**(Suppl 6): 160S–198S.
Baglin TP, Keeling DM, Watson HG, British Committee for Standards in Haematology. Guidelines on oral anticoagulation (warfarin): third edition – 2005 update. *Br J Haematol* 2006; **132:** 277–285.
Link KP. The discovery of Dicumarol and its sequels. *Circulation* 1959; **19:** 97–107.

Chapter 2

Stroke prevention, atrial fibrillation and indications for warfarin

Dr P Rose

Learning outcomes

- **Atrial fibrillation as a risk factor for stroke**
- **The clinical indications for warfarin and the therapeutic target international normalised ratio (INR) (British Society for Haematology guidelines)**

The number of patients requiring long-term oral anticoagulant treatment for primary and secondary prevention of stroke in patients with atrial fibrillation (AF) continues to increase. Currently, AF represents the most common reason for oral anticoagulation in the UK, accounting for up to 70% of the one million patients on oral anticoagulation.

Evidence for oral anticoagulation therapy

A simple model for deciding to treat with oral anticoagulation based on available evidence can be expressed by the equation:

net benefit = the absolute risk x the relative risk – harm

Adverse risk factors for oral anticoagulant therapy are often factors that, paradoxically, make patients most at risk of developing strokes, such as increasing age, diabetes and congestive heart disease. The level of evidence favouring anticoagulation can be graded, based on current published findings. However, a more refined approach should take into account the patient's specific clinical history, previous stability and adverse events on anticoagulants. A method to assess the patient's risk of bleeding has been reported by Beyth, with increased risk associated with a history of previous stroke, gastrointestinal bleeding, a specific comorbid condition, raised serum creatinine, a low haematocrit level and diabetes. These parameters can be used to identify patients who are at a low, intermediate or high risk of bleeding events.

Evidence to suggest that oral anticoagulation is of benefit for patients with AF has accumulated over the last 20 years. The results of pooled data from five randomised, controlled trials of primary prevention, started in the 1980s, demonstrated a 68% risk reduction for patients treated with warfarin. Virtually no increase in the frequency of major bleeding was attributed to warfarin in these trials. In interpreting these data, it should be pointed out that many of the trials had large exclusion criteria and, as such, the patients included were less likely to run into problems with adverse events. Furthermore, the quality of anticoagulation and the intensity of follow-up reported in the trials is often difficult to reproduce in routine clinical practice.

In recent years, studies using the direct thrombin inhibitor ximelagatran have shown this to be a highly effective anticoagulant agent when given as a fixed dose without laboratory monitoring. A large meta-analysis comparing stroke prevention with aspirin, warfarin and ximelagatran in AF patients confirmed the superiority of this agent over aspirin and found it to be as effective as adjusted-dose warfarin, with a lower risk of bleeding. Unfortunately, this agent was withdrawn by AstraZeneca, as a very small number of patients were reported to have serious liver toxicity. There are, however, new direct thrombin and anti-Xa inhibitors under evaluation, both in the setting of venous thromboembolic disease and AF, which are likely to have a major impact on anticoagulant practice in the next few years.

What is the risk of stroke with AF?

The fact that AF is a risk factor for stroke was well demonstrated in the Framingham Heart Study. A fivefold increase in stroke rate was identified in patients with AF, which increases with age, such that 25% of all strokes in those aged 80–89 were associated with AF. Furthermore, the death rate was significantly raised and chronic disability was higher in patients with AF who had strokes than in those with sinus rhythm. The true prevalence of AF in the UK is difficult to determine and may be higher than reported, since AF can be transient or paroxysmal and many patients are asymptomatic. This was well illustrated in a UK study, in which only 76% of patients with AF had the diagnosis recorded in their medical records. Another community survey identified that only 30% of patients with AF ever presented to hospital practice. These studies also looked at the number of patients receiving anticoagulant treatment. There has been a major improvement in the uptake of oral anticoagulation in the UK in the last few years, particularly following the National Institute for Health and Clinical Excellence (NICE) guidance on the management of AF and the recommendations from the National Patient Safety Agency on anticoagulant therapy.

How effective is warfarin in preventing strokes?

It has been estimated that to prevent one stroke using warfarin as primary prevention in AF, 32 patients would require anticoagulation therapy. For patients who have had a previous stroke, 12 patients would need to be treated to prevent one further event. This compares very favourably, however, with antihypertensive therapy and secondary prevention with statins.

There is evidence that adjusted-dose warfarin versus placebo is strongly associated with a lower incidence of stroke. For all patients with AF receiving adjusted-dose warfarin, there is an association with a higher incidence of major bleeding events, compared with placebo. However, there is no significant association between adjusted-dose warfarin and the incidence of haemorrhagic stroke and other bleeding events for patients with no previous stroke or transient ischaemic attacks. Significantly, adjusted-dose warfarin is associated with a decreased likelihood of severe or fatal stroke compared with low-dose warfarin and with a significant reduction in ischaemic stroke compared with aspirin. Adjusted-dose warfarin is also associated with a higher instance of major bleeding events compared with aspirin but not compared with low-dose warfarin regimens. Overall, warfarin is the most effective agent for stroke reduction in patients with AF. It is particularly effective for patients with a previous history of stroke or transient ischaemic attack, patients with hypertension or diabetes, patients over 75 years of age and patients with impaired left ventricular function. Currently, there is no role for low-dose warfarin regimens. There is also no clear evidence that oral anticoagulation in the absence of AF prevents recurrent strokes.

In addition, there is no evidence that old age alone is a contraindication to warfarin therapy. Warfarin requirements will be much less in the very elderly and a detailed assessment relating to compliance is important before considering anticoagulant treatment.

British Society for Haematology recommendations and therapeutic target international normalised ratio

Non-rheumatic AF

Studies looking at low-intensity oral anticoagulation in AF have been compared with dose-adjusted warfarin anticoagulation in high-risk patients by the Stroke Prevention in Atrial Fibrillation (SPAF) 3 trial. In this study, a low-intensity anticoagulant arm to achieve an international normalised ratio (INR) of 1.2–1.5 plus aspirin 325 mg was compared with dose-adjusted oral anticoagulation to achieve an INR of between 2 and 3. The stroke/embolic rate per year, however, was 7.9% in the low-dose and aspirin arm, compared with only 1.9% in the dose-adjusted oral anticoagulant arm. It is, therefore, difficult to justify this approach. Furthermore, in a primary care-based prevention study of arterial thromboembolism in patients with non-rheumatic AF with a low risk, major haemorrhage occurred with standard anticoagulation at a rate of 0.5 per 100 patient-years, compared with aspirin at 1.4 per 100 patient-years and with low-dose anticoagulants from 1.4 per 100 patient-years. It should be remembered that aspirin is also associated with increased risk of bleeding and is not necessarily a safer option.

The British Society for Haematology recommendations for oral anticoagulation in patients with non-rheumatic AF are:
- Patients with no risk factors under the age of 65 should receive aspirin 150 mg daily
- Patients with risk factors should receive warfarin to achieve a target INR of 2.5
- Patients over 65 with additional risk factors should receive warfarin if there are no serious adverse risk factors.

Mechanical and bioprosthetic valves

The distribution of mechanical and bioprosthetic valves in the UK differs according to age. In general, older patients receive bioprosthetic valves, while younger patients receive longer-lasting mechanical valves. In one study, 52% of patients with aortic valves – either tissue or mechanical valves – survived ten years, during which time 42%

had an adverse event of haemorrhage or thrombosis, with no difference in the outcome of patients who receive mechanical or bioprosthetic valves. For patients with bioprosthetic valves in the aortic position, the value of subsequent oral anticoagulation is minimal. Currently, a maximum period of three months' anticoagulation therapy is commonly administered to achieve an INR of 2.5.

The need for three months of anticoagulation therapy following a mitral bioprosthetic valve is much clearer. However, for any patients with bioprosthetic valves who have AF, lifelong oral anticoagulation will be needed. Furthermore, patients who have had a history of systemic emboli or cardiac thrombus should also receive lifelong anticoagulation.

For mechanical valves, higher levels of anticoagulation have been routinely used. More recently, it has been suggested that the position of the valve and the nature of the mechanical valve may have some bearing on the level of anticoagulant prophylaxis needed. The thrombotic risk is higher with mitral valve replacements, although more recent mechanical valves are less thrombogenic than some of the older valves. The current recommendation is for a target INR of 3.5, with lifelong duration for older mechanical valves (for example, Starr-Edwards or Bjork-Shiley). This is based on results published in 1995 by Cannegieter *et al*, demonstrating increased thrombotic events occurring with INR values less than 2.5 and increased haemorrhagic events occurring with INR values greater than 5. For current valve replacements, a target INR of 3 is reasonable in the mitral position, with a target INR of 2.5 for bileaflet valves in the aortic position.

A number of studies have looked at the use of oral anticoagulation in conjunction with aspirin and dipyridamole for patients with mechanical heart valves. Varying doses of aspirin and dipyridamole have been used; a combination of aspirin 660 mg and dipyridamole 150 mg resulted in 24.7% of cases having a major bleed, when combined with an INR range of 3–4.5. This contrasts with an INR range of 2.5–3.5, combined with aspirin 100 mg daily, which resulted in 1.1% major bleeds and only 1.3% thromboembolic events per year. Overall, from six major studies reported to date, the risk of bleeding is too high to currently recommend this approach. Additional antiplatelet agents should be reserved for patients with embolic events despite adequate oral anticoagulation.

Venous thrombosis

Patients with deep vein thrombosis (DVT) require anticoagulation to prevent extension and embolisation of clots. The duration of therapy, however, is debatable. Venous thromboembolic disease is best considered as a chronic disorder. The longer-term sequelae of postphlebitic syndrome and chronic venous ulceration are commonly seen in primary care but are less well recognised in hospital medicine. The recommended duration of oral anticoagulation for proximal vein thrombosis is based on two studies.

First, Levine *et al* in 1995 reported that the recurrent rate would be 6% following four weeks of oral anticoagulation, compared with 0.9% with three months of oral anticoagulation. Schulman *et al*, in the same year, reported the recurrence rates for DVT to be 18.1% with six weeks' anticoagulation, compared with 9.5% with six months' anticoagulation. Current recommendations are that an INR target value of 2.5 is indicated and oral anticoagulation should be continued for six months for patients with a proximal vein thrombosis.

In 1999, a study by Kearon and colleagues compared the recurrence rate of patients with a first idiopathic venous thrombosis given three months' oral anticoagulation followed by placebo, with that of those receiving continuous warfarin (mean follow-up ten months). The recurrence rate was 27.4% per patient-year in those receiving three months' oral anticoagulation and placebo, compared with 1.3% per patient-year with continuous warfarin. Warfarin resulted in a 95% reduction in the risk of recurrent venous thromboembolism. This study was discontinued early in view of the obvious benefit in terms of longer oral anticoagulation. Further studies have since shown the recurrence rate of unprovoked DVT of around 10% within 12 months, and 30% within five years, of stopping anticoagulant therapy.

For patients in whom there is an obvious precipitating factor, such as post-surgery, a shorter period of anticoagulation of three months is recommended. For patients in whom the post-surgical DVT is confined to the calf, six weeks of treatment has been shown to be effective. It is, therefore, necessary at the start of anticoagulation to define the extent of the clot and to identify any precipitating factors. Where there are continuing risk factors, a longer duration of anticoagulation should be considered.

Thrombophilia screening

Thrombophilia screening is increasingly performed for patients with a history of venous thrombosis. For patients with one thrombotic event, there is no evidence to suggest that a longer duration of anticoagulation is necessary if they are heterozygous for factor V Leiden, prothrombin gene mutation, protein C or protein S deficiency.

Where there are combinations of thrombotic risk factors, long-term anticoagulation would be considered. Long-term anticoagulation would also be recommended for patients with recurrent venous thromboembolic events, where there are no short-term risk factors to account for the event, or when there is a strong family history of venous thrombosis.

Summary

- Currently, atrial fibrillation (AF) represents the most common reason for oral anticoagulation in the UK, accounting for up to 70% of the one million patients on these drugs.
- The results of pooled data from five randomised, controlled trials of primary prevention demonstrated a 68% risk reduction for patients treated with warfarin.
- In recent years, studies using the direct thrombin inhibitor ximelagatran have shown this to be a highly effective anticoagulant agent when given as a fixed dose without laboratory monitoring. A large meta-analysis comparing stroke prevention with aspirin, warfarin and ximelagatran in AF patients confirmed the superiority of this agent over aspirin and found it to be as effective as adjusted-dose warfarin, with a lower risk of bleeding. Unfortunately, this agent was withdrawn by AstraZeneca, as a very small number of patients were reported to have serious liver toxicity. There are, however, new direct thrombin and anti-Xa inhibitors under evaluation, both in the setting of venous thromboembolic disease and AF, which are likely to have a major impact on anticoagulant practice in the next few years.

- The Framingham Heart Study identified a fivefold increase in stroke rate for patients with AF, which increases with age, such that 25% of all strokes in those aged 80–89 were associated with AF.
- It has been estimated that to prevent one stroke using warfarin as primary prevention in AF patients, 32 patients would need to be anticoagulated.
- The British Society for Haematology recommendations for oral anticoagulation for patients with non-rheumatic AF are:
  - Patients with no risk factors under the age of 65 should receive 150 mg of aspirin per day
  - Patients with risk factors should receive warfarin to achieve a target international normalised ratio of 2.5
  - Patients over 65 with additional risk factors should receive warfarin if there are no serious adverse risk factors.
- For all mechanical heart valves, a target INR of 3 is recommended and additional antiplatelet agents should be reserved for patients with embolic events despite adequate oral anticoagulation.
- Current recommendations for patients with a proximal vein thrombosis are an INR target value of 2.5 and oral anticoagulation to be continued for six months.
- Long-term anticoagulation is recommended for patients with recurrent venous thromboembolic events where there are no short-term risk factors to account for the event.

Further reading

Beyth RJ, Quinn LM, Landerfield S. Prospective evaluation of an index for predicting risk of major bleeding in outpatients treated with warfarin. *Am J Med* 1998; **105:** 91–99.

Atrial Fibrillation Investigators. Risk factors for stroke and efficacy of anti-thrombotic therapy in atrial fibrillation. Analysis of pooled data from five randomised trials. *Arch Intern Med* 1994; **154:** 1445–1457.

Wolf PA, Abbot RD, Kannal WB. Atrial fibrillation as an independent risk factor for stroke: The Framingham Study. *Stroke* 1991; **22:** 983–988.

Sudlow M, Rodgers H, Henry RA *et al.* Population based study of use of anticoagulants among patients with atrial fibrillation in the community. *BMJ* 1997; **314:** 1529–1530.

Lip GYH, Golding GJ, Razir M *et al.* A survey of atrial fibrillation in general practice. The West Birmingham Atrial Fibrillation Project. *Br J Gen Pract* 1997; **47:** 285–289.

British Committee for Standards in Haematology (BCSH). Guidelines on oral anticoagulation: third edition. *Br J Haematol* 1998; **101:** 374–387.

Stroke Prevention in Atrial Fibrillation Investigations. Adjusted dose warfarin versus low intensity, fixed dose warfarin plus aspirin for high risk atrial fibrillation. *Lancet* 1996; **348:** 633–638.

Peterseim DS, Cen YY, Cheruvu S *et al.* Long-term outcome after biological versus mechanical aortic valve replacements in 841 patients. *J Thorac Cardiovasc Surg* 1999; **117:** 890–897.

Cannegieter S, Rosendall F, Wintzen A *et al.* Optimal oral anticoagulant therapy in patients with mechanical valves. *N Engl J Med* 1995; **333:** 11–12.

Turpie AGG. Valvular heart disease and heart valve prostheses. In: Poller L, Hirsh J (eds). *Oral anticoagulants.* London: Hodder Arnold, 1996: 143–149.

Levine M, Hirsh J, Gent M *et al.* Optimal duration of oral anticoagulant therapy: a randomised trial comparing four weeks with three months of warfarin in patients with proximal vein thrombosis. *Thromb Haemostas* 1995; **74:** 606–611.

Schulman S, Rhedin A, Lindmarker P *et al.* A comparison of six weeks with six months of oral anticoagulation therapy after a first episode of venous thromboembolism. *N Engl J Med* 1995; **332:** 1661–1665.

Kearon C, Gent M, Hirsh J *et al.* A comparison of three months anticoagulation with extended anticoagulation for a first episode of idiopathic venous thromboembolism. *N Engl J Med* 1999; **340:** 901–907.

Walker I, Greaves M, Preston FE on behalf of the Haemostasis and Thrombosis Task Force. Investigation and management of heritable thrombophilia. *Br J Haematol* 2001; **114:** 512–528.

Baglin TP, Keeling DM, Watson HG, British Committee for Standards in Haematology. Guidelines on oral anticoagulation (warfarin): third edition – 2005 update. *Br J Haematol* 2006; **132:** 277–285.

Lip GY, Edwards SJ. Stroke prevention with aspirin, warfarin and ximelagatran in patients with non-valvular atrial fibrillation: a systemic review and meta-analysis. *Thromb Res* 2006; **118:** 321–333.

Chapter 3

Anticoagulant point-of-care testing (POCT)

Mr C Gardiner

Professor SJ Machin

Learning outcomes

- **International normalised ratio (INR) measurement and thromboplastins**
- **Point-of-care testing and evidence for clinical effectiveness**

Thromboplastins

The prothrombin time (PT) assessment uses a thromboplastin – an extract of tissue factor (TF) – to accelerate the clotting time of recalcified plasma. It is sensitive to changes in the levels of the vitamin K-dependent factors II, VII and X and so is used almost universally to control oral anticoagulant therapy. A variety of sources of TF have been used to prepare thromboplastin, including human, bovine and rabbit brain, human placenta and, more recently, recombinant human and rabbit preparations relipidated with natural or synthetic phospholipids. Commercial thromboplastins may also contain buffers, preservatives and heparin neutralisers, such as polybrene.

The prothrombin time ratio (PTR) was an attempt to compare patient results with a normal value for individuals not taking oral anticoagulants. It is derived as follows. Each laboratory establishes a normal reference range for each reagent and technique employed, using samples from at least 20 healthy adults. From this, the geometric mean normal PT (MNPT) is calculated so that the PTR may be calculated:

PTR = test PT/MNPT

However, it has long been recognised that PTRs performed on the same sample show poor agreement between different laboratories and that this is due to a number of pre-test and analytical variables (Table 3.1, page 14), the most important of which is the type of thromboplastin used. This inconsistency could easily lead to the incorrect dosing of patients – with potentially life-threatening consequences.

The international normalised ratio

The international normalised ratio (INR) was developed in the 1980s, in an attempt to standardise the PT for use in the control of long-term oral anticoagulation. Each thromboplastin is assigned an international sensitivity index (ISI) by the manufacturer, which reflects the reagent sensitivity to the reduced levels of factors II and VII, due to oral anticoagulation.

The INR may be defined as the prothrombin ratio that would have been obtained using the first primary international reference preparation (IRP), arbitrarily assigned an ISI of 1.0, using a manual tube tilt technique. It is calculated as follows:

$$INR = (patient\ PT/MNPT)^{ISI}$$

It is important that the ISI and MNPT are calculated for each new batch of thromboplastin with each coagulometer used. ISI calibration is discussed in detail in the WHO Expert Committee on Biological Standardisation (1999) recommendations. There is a consensus of opinion that, wherever possible, backed by external quality assessment (EQA) data, low ISI thromboplastins (between 1.0–1.4) should be used for INR determination, as the higher ISI reagents are associated with a high degree of imprecision. This is of major clinical importance, since the width of the therapeutic range diminishes progressively with increasing INR. Furthermore, the use of high ISI reagents may give less dependable INR values during the induction period of oral anticoagulation and in poorly stabilised patients.

Table 3.1. Factors affecting the prothrombin time

Pre-test variables
- Citrate concentration
- Blood collection tube type
- Sample activation due to poor venepuncture technique
- Severe anaemia or polycythaemia
- Under- or overfilling of blood collection tube
- Prolonged storage of samples
- Heparin contamination from indwelling catheters or intravenous lines
- Clinical state (impaired liver function, heparin therapy)
- Lupus anticoagulant
- Interfering substances (hyperlipidaemia, severe icterus)

Analytical variables
- Thromboplastin source
- Coagulometer effects
- Analysis temperature
- Calcium concentration

Point-of-care testing (near-patient testing) INR measurement

A current estimate of the number of patients on oral anticoagulation is unavailable; however, it is likely that over one million people in the UK currently take warfarin. This number is estimated to increase by approximately 15% per year. The increased use of warfarin is largely related to an aging population and newer indications for long-term anticoagulation, particularly atrial fibrillation, but also primary prevention of ischaemic heart disease and long-term prevention of recurrent venous thromboembolism. The traditional model of long-term anticoagulant care involves repeated attendance at a hospital-based anticoagulation clinic, with PT/INR testing usually performed at a centralised hospital laboratory. However, the increase in patient referrals has prompted the investigation of several new models of patient care, involving various degrees of decentralisation. Many of these rely on point-of-care testing (POCT), also known as near-patient testing (NPT), which may be defined as testing performed in close proximity to patients. The geographical location is a prime factor in deciding the degree of decentralisation employed. In inner city areas, blood collection and dosing may be performed in a nurse-led clinic, whereas in rural areas patient self-testing is more appropriate, with either centralised dosing by a healthcare professional, or patient self-management (the patient performs both testing and dosing). The patient training on the use of such devices needs to follow nationally agreed guidelines and recommendations.

There are several devices available for POCT coagulation testing. These fall broadly into one of two types:

● Devices designed for professional use, primarily for non-laboratory hospital staff
● Devices intended for use by patients themselves.

The former devices may allow tests other than INR to be performed on the same instrument – for example, activated partial thromboplastin time (APTT) or activated clotting time (ACT) – and may permit the use of more than one sample type. They have large electronic memories and relatively complex data management systems suitable for multi-user, multipatient use, whereas the latter devices perform only PT/INR testing with more basic software, with the emphasis on ease of use. Devices for POCT

Table 3.2. Requirements for POCT devices for use in primary care and patient self-testing

● The INR result must be accurate and reproducible
● The result must be clearly displayed
● A suitable quality control (QC) package should ensure the validity of results
● There must be adequate capacity for result storage. This will vary depending on whether it is intended for single patient or clinic use
● Patient and QC results should be readily distinguishable
● There should be an output for data to be printed or sent to a computer
● Devices must have a small sample volume requirement (<50 ml)
● There should be no requirement for accurate blood volume measurement
● They must be compatible with capillary or venous blood
● The sample application point must be easily accessible for elderly patients (many of whom may have poor flexibility)
● They must be simple to use and not require a high degree of dexterity
● They should be small enough to be easily portable and, ideally, hand-held and low in weight
● Each device must bear a *Conformité Européenne* (CE) mark

monitoring of oral anticoagulation must satisfy certain requirements (Table 3.2, page 15) in order to be suitable for primary care and patient self-testing.

The available POCT devices

At the time of writing, there are three POCT devices intended solely for use in monitoring oral anticoagulation, either by healthcare professionals or patients: the CoaguChek® XS (Roche Diagnostics, UK), shown in Figure 3.1, the ProTime® (International Technidyne Corp, USA), shown in Figure 3.2 and the INRatio™ (HemoSense Inc, USA) shown in Figure 3.3. All three have received a *Conformité Européenne* (CE) mark, which is now mandatory for all *in vitro* diagnostic devices. Although all three devices measure the PT on native capillary or venous blood, each uses a different measuring principle. The CoaguChek® XS performs an electrochemical measurement of the PT using a recombinant human thromboplastin reagent and a peptide substrate. Application of sample leads to activation of coagulation by the thromboplastin and results in thrombin generation. Thrombin cleaves the substrate into a residual peptide and electrochemically active phenylenediamine, thereby generating an electrochemical signal. The time elapsed from addition of sample to signal generation is used to calculate the INR value. The ProTime® optically detects the motion of the blood sample, which is pumped back and forth within the capillaries of the test strip containing freeze-dried thromboplastin, until clot formation stops blood flow, and the endpoint is recorded. The INRatio™ uses test strips containing thromboplastin in which clot formation is detected by a change in the electrical impedance of the blood sample that occurs when fibrinogen is converted to fibrin.

Two further devices suitable for professional monitoring of PT/INR in primary care are available: The CoaguChek® XS Plus is a professional version of the CoaguChek® XS. It uses the same measuring principle, but it has more QC and data handling options, positive patient identification, a bidirectional interface and storage capacity for up to 500 results. The Hemochron® Jr Signature+ (International Technidyne Corp) uses the same measuring principle as the ProTime®, but has a data storage module, an RS-232 interface, numeric patient identification, and operator identification and storage for up to 400 patient test results and 400 QC results.

POCT evaluation

As with all *in vitro* diagnostic equipment, POCT equipment should be thoroughly evaluated prior to clinical implementation to ensure that reliable results are consistently obtained. In the UK, this was previously performed on by the Centre for Evidence-based Purchasing of the Department of Health. These evaluations were full national evaluations, under highly controlled conditions in the laboratory or clinic, using just one or two experienced operators. Although no specific guidelines for the INR calibration of POCT devices are currently available, it is accepted that INR calibration should be performed by the manufacturers using the same procedure as conventional laboratory systems. ISI and MNPT calibration are as performed by the manufacturers and cannot be altered by the user. Independent attempts to verify the manufacturers' INR calibrations have been performed in a few expert laboratories using the World Health

Organization IRP, but this is not generally feasible or necessary. For this reason, POCT devices' PT and INRs should be compared with those obtained with at least two other reference systems selected from instruments and reagents that have previously been widely validated. The thromboplastins selected must have an ISI for the particular endpoint detection method used. Most POCT instruments operate on whole blood, and these thromboplastin reagents may behave differently from some of those used in routine hospital laboratories. No formal evaluation service now exists in the UK, so the onus is on the end-user to ensure that a POCT device gives safe, accurate results.

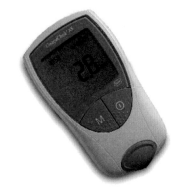

Figure 3.1. The CoaguChek® XS device

Assessment process

Inter-instrument variability may be assessed by testing approximately six normal samples, and 12–18 oral anticoagulant samples on each of three different instruments, using a single cartridge batch. Test-strip between-batch variability is tested using one instrument with three different lot numbers of test cartridges, using approximately six normal samples, and 12–18 oral anticoagulant samples.

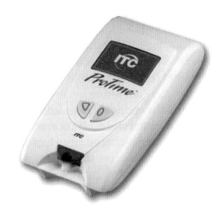

Figure 3.2. The ProTime® device

In instruments that allow the use of lyophilised plasma/whole blood QC preparations, within-day and total imprecision testing may be assessed by testing three replicates of each QC preparation over five separate days. Within-day imprecision is obtained by calculating the mean percentage coefficient of variation (%CV) for day, while total imprecision is found by calculating the overall %CV. If the instrument does not allow the use of lyophilised QC preparations, within-day imprecision may be determined by testing five individuals in triplicate and calculating the mean %CV.

If a laboratory evaluation shows the instrument performance to be satisfactory, an operational evaluation 'in the field'

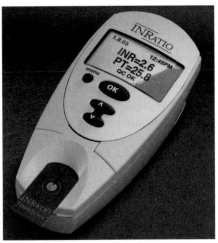

Figure 3.3. The INRatio™ device

Table 3.3. Requirements for primary care point-of-care testing (POCT) for oral anticoagulation control

Cost-benefit analysis

● The need for POCT must be demonstrated (it may be more expensive than the existing hospital system)

● The local haematology department and consultant in charge should be involved

● Costs should be pre-assessed for all running costs and overheads – including training, support, quality control (QC) or quality assurance (QA) and replacement

● The POCT device should be satisfactorily evaluated (full Medicines and Healthcare products Regulatory Agency [MHRA] and operational evaluations)

● Registration should be made for external QA (UK National External Quality Assessment Service schemes are most appropriate)

Risk management

● The risks associated with the use of the POCT instrument and interpretation of the results must be considered

Health and safety

● Procedures for disinfection of the POCT device and disposal of the consumables should be established

Training

● A structured teaching and assessment programme is necessary

● Consideration should be given to who will perform the training

● The local NHS trust haematologist should be contacted

● A standard operating procedure should be produced, taking into account local guidelines. This should be written to the standard required by Clinical Pathology Accreditation (UK) Ltd or an equivalent body

● Safe INR limits should be agreed, outside of which the haematology department is informed

Operation

● Consideration should be given to who will perform the testing

● Only named staff/patients who have received satisfactory training should perform any testing

Recording of information

● All patient test results and QC data must be recorded and stored safely

● Maintenance and repairs should be recorded in a logbook

(under the conditions most likely to be encountered in normal everyday use), may be indicated. This should involve the healthcare staff or patients who will be using the instrument. In addition to analytical performance, this evaluation should also assess the user acceptability of the device

There is a large number of recently published evaluations of INR measurements in POCT settings, including testing by healthcare professionals in hospitals and primary care, patient self-testing with centralised dosing, and patient self-testing and management. Some studies simply compare the POCT INR measurement with a centralised laboratory measurement, whereas others – particularly the self-testing/management studies – have compared the clinical outcome in terms of the time spent in the therapeutic range or the frequency of bleeding or thrombotic events during the study. On the basis of the published literature, the performance of POCT devices is comparable with conventional laboratory testing. Perhaps more unexpected is the repeated finding that patient self-testing/patient self-management (PST/PSM) is superior to conventional hospital management in terms of clinical outcome. This is thought to be due, at least in part, to more frequent testing (usually at weekly or fortnightly intervals), better patient understanding and improved compliance.

The potential benefits of monitoring oral anticoagulation therapy in primary care are well documented. Ever-increasing numbers of patients are placing demands on hospital anticoagulant clinics in terms of time, money and space. This inevitably leads to longer waiting times for patients, who already suffer considerable disruption as a result of anticoagulation. Practice nurse-led testing or patient self-testing reduces waiting times and travelling distances (especially in rural areas). Although self-testing has been reported as less cost-effective than routine clinic care, the assessment looked only at the direct costs to the NHS and did not take into account elements such as transport for the patient and lost patient working time. The uptake in trials of PST/PSM in the UK has typically been highly variable, prompting suggestions that self-monitoring of oral anticoagulation therapy is suitable for only a minority of patients. However, a recent study has shown that almost half of patients receiving long-term oral anticoagulation will elect for self-monitoring if offered at the start of treatment.

There are several important considerations to be made before implementing POCT in a primary care setting, as outlined in Table 3.3, page 18.

Conclusions

The future management/organisation of oral anticoagulation control is difficult to reliably predict, particularly as the number of patients receiving oral anticoagulation is increasing by approximately 10% per year. The manufacturers are producing smaller, lighter hand-held devices; in future these may have the capacity to recommend appropriate dosage changes. Published clinical guidelines must be carefully followed by healthcare professionals and individual patients, with the hope that government or private health insurers will recognise the need for financial reimbursement to purchase instruments and disposable test strips. The test strips have been available on the Drug Tariff in the UK since May 2003, although some primary care trusts have shown reluctance to allow their prescription. 2008 has seen the first licences for the new generation of oral antithrombotic compounds that do not require regular laboratory monitoring. The uptake of these drugs over the next few years will have a huge influence on the future of oral anticoagulation.

Summary

- The prothrombin time (PT) uses a thromboplastin – an extract of tissue factor (TF) – to accelerate the clotting time of recalcified plasma.
- The geometric mean normal PT (MNPT) is calculated so that the prothrombin time ratio (PTR) may be calculated as test PT/MNPT.
- Each thromboplastin is assigned an international sensitivity index (ISI) by the manufacturer, which reflects the sensitivity of the reagent to the reduced levels of factors II and VII.
- The international normalised ratio (INR) = (patient PT/MNPT)^{ISI}.
- Point-of-care testing (POCT), also known as near-patient testing, may be defined as testing performed in close proximity to patients.
- POCT equipment should be thoroughly evaluated before clinical implementation to ensure that reliable results are consistently obtained.
- It is the responsibility of the end-user to determine the suitability of POCT devices for clinical practice.
- The requirements for POCT devices in primary care include the following:
- INR must be accurate and reproducible, with the result clearly displayed
- It must need only a small sample, with no accurate blood volume required
- There must be adequate and appropriate storage
- It must be simple to use and portable.

Further reading
Briggs C, Guthrie D, Hyde K *et al.* British Committee for Standards in Haematology (BCSH) General Haematology Task Force. Guidelines for point-of-care testing: haematology (2008). http://www.bcshguidelines.com
Cromheecke ME, Levi M, Colly LP *et al.* Oral anticoagulation self-management and management by a specialist anticoagulation clinic: a randomised cross-over comparison. *Lancet* 2000; **356:** 97–102.
Connock M, Stevens C, Fry-Smith A *et al.* Clinical effectiveness and cost-effectiveness of different models of managing long-term oral anticoagulation therapy: a systematic review and economic modelling. *Health Technol Assess* 2007; **11:** 1–86.
Fitzmaurice DA, Gardiner C, Kitchen S *et al.* An evidence-based review and guidelines for patient self-testing and management of oral anticoagulation. *Br J Haematol* 2005; **131:** 156–165.
Heneghan C, Alonso-Coello P, Garcia-Alamino JM *et al.* P. Self-monitoring of oral anticoagulation: a systematic review and meta-analysis. *Lancet* 2006; **367:** 404–411.
Tripodi A, Chantarangul V, Clerici M, Negri B, Mannucci PM. Determination of the International Sensitivity Index of a new near-patient testing device to monitor oral anticoagulant therapy. Overview on the assessment of conformity to the calibration model. *Thrombosis Haemostasis* 1997; **78:** 855–858.
WHO Expert Committee on Biological Standardisation. *Technical Report Series 889.* Geneva: World Health Organization, 1999.

All published reports are freely available at
http://www.pasa.nhs.uk/PASAWeb/NHSprocurement/CEP

Chapter 4

Internal quality control and external quality assessment of the INR using POC monitors

Mrs DP Kitchen

Dr S Kitchen

Professor ID Walker

Learning outcome

● **Quality issues in relation to the determination of an international normalised ratio (INR), using point-of-care testing coagulometers, including internal quality control and external quality assessment**

Quality assurance (QA) is an overall term that may be used to describe all measures that are taken to ensure the reliability of testing and reporting. This includes the collection of a valid sample from the patient, analysis of the specimen and the accurate recording of results, as well as interpretation of the results.

Internal quality control (IQC) and external quality assessment (EQA) are two distinct yet complementary components of the QA programme. IQC is used to establish whether the particular technique is performing consistently over a period of time. It is, therefore, deployed to ensure day-to-day consistency. EQA is used to identify the degree of agreement between one centre's results and those obtained by other centres. In large EQA schemes, retrospective analysis of results obtained by participating centres permits the identification of poor individual performance and also provides information about results with different methods.

Internal quality control

IQC is used to establish whether a particular method is giving consistent results on different occasions. The expression quality control is commonly used to describe the set of procedures used to check that the results of investigations are reliable enough to be released to assist clinical decision-making; for example, in the monitoring of oral anticoagulant therapy. Quality control procedures should be applied in a way that ensures immediate and constant control of result generation. The quality of results obtained is

influenced by many factors, which include the following:
● Appropriate sample collection and handling
● Selection of a suitable technique
● Maintenance of up-to-date standard operational procedures
● Adequate records and reporting system for results.

In addition, the quality of results obtained in routine practice is highly dependent on the selection, training and motivation of suitable personnel.

IQC is particularly useful for identifying the degree of precision of a particular technique, precision being the degree of agreement among repeat measurements on one sample. It is important to recognise that a precise technique is not necessarily accurate, accuracy being a measure of the closeness of an estimated value to the true value.

Electronic IQC

Determination of international normalised ratios (INRs) with point-of-care (POC) monitors involves insertion of an individual test strip or cartridge into the monitor. The addition of a blood sample results in reconstitution of the dried thromboplastin reagent on the test strip or cartridge, initiating the clotting reaction. Clot formation is detected by the POC monitor and converted into an INR value. For a number of POC monitors, electronic IQC is available. With these monitors, an electronic device is inserted into the monitor in place of the test strip and blood sample. A signal is produced which tests the optical and/or electronic system within the POC monitor. A result is usually displayed as an apparent clotting time, mimicking the analysis of a blood sample. Although this type of IQC can confirm that some parts of the analytical process are performing adequately, it is not sufficient as the only form of IQC. It does not indicate whether a batch of test strips has been stored and handled appropriately, and whether the batch is meeting its specification. To confirm that a group of test strips are suitable for testing patients' blood samples, a liquid control, which can be tested and will clot in a similar way to a blood sample, is required.

Inbuilt IQC

At least three manufacturers of POC materials produce INR test strips which have an inbuilt IQC function. Test strips for the ProTime® monitor (International Technidyne Corp, USA) have five capillaries down which the blood sample flows. Three of these capillaries are used for replicate INR measurement of the patient's blood. The outer left and outer right capillaries contain control material, which is reconstituted by the patient's blood. An alternative ProTime® test strip has three capillaries (two IQC and one patient test). The ProTime® monitor indicates whether the IQC results are acceptable, but does not display an INR result for the IQC. Test strips for the INRatio™ monitor also have inbuilt IQC, but in this case the INRatio™ monitor displays an INR value for the IQC material. The CoaguChek® XS and CoaguChek® XS Plus devices have an on-board strip integrity check. This is a chemical reaction that occurs alongside the patient's sample clotting but is a chemical cleavage which is measured by the change in electrical impedance. These two devices indicate that the test strip has passed the integrity check by showing a tick icon on the screen, which allows testing to proceed.

As for the electronic IQC described above, inbuilt IQC, whether included in the test strips or on-board the monitor, is not acceptable as the only means of IQC. To be adequate, IQC must include analysis of a liquid control tested in the same way as patient samples and with results displayed as INR. This is a difficult area, as some POC monitors do not provide a liquid IQC sample.

Liquid IQC

Some manufacturers of POC monitors and test strips for INR determination have control materials available for the purpose of IQC for their systems. Some manufacturers provide a vial of lyophilised plasma together with a sealed pipette that contains the required amount of diluent. One example takes the form of a small flexible plastic dropper unit containing lyophilised plasma and a fragile sealed ampoule of diluent (Figure 4.1). Gentle pressure crushes the ampoule, releasing the diluent to dissolve the plasma. The crushed glass ampoule remains safely within the strong plastic dropper. After a fixed reconstitution period, the plasma is squeezed through a dropper onto a test strip and analysed as though it were a patient blood sample. Other commercial IQC samples contain lyophilised whole blood with reconstitution fluid provided. All the materials required are provided and no laboratory facility or equipment is required for analysis, making them particularly suitable for POC sites.

The frequency of analysis of liquid IQC should depend on the number of patient samples analysed. If a small group of tests (fewer than ten) is performed within a four-hour period, a single IQC analysis should be included. If a larger group of tests is performed over the same day, IQC samples should be included at the beginning and end of testing. If an unexpected patient result is obtained, it is useful to test an IQC sample at that time to confirm that the test system has remained in control.

In some cases, IQC samples with a range of normal and abnormal results are available. For monitoring coumarin anticoagulants, the most suitable IQC samples would have results within the therapeutic range (INR 2.0–4.0). For each IQC sample, there should be a target range within which results are acceptable. If a result of an IQC sample lies outside the target range, a second sample should be tested. If the second result is also out of range, patient testing should be suspended until the cause has been identified and corrected. The storage conditions of the test strips and IQC material

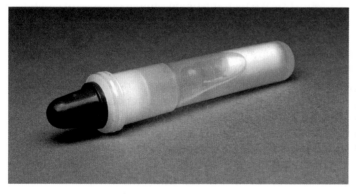

Figure 4.1. Internal quality control sample for some point-of-care testing monitors. Diluent and lyophilised plasma are contained within a strong plastic dropper, separated by fragile glass and mixed after gentle pressure crushes the glass

should be checked, as well as the performance of the monitor. This may involve the manufacturer of the test system. Manufacturers normally provide acceptable limits for results of their QC materials. In some cases, their limits may be inappropriately wide; sometimes as much as ±1.0 INR units of a value (for example, target INR 3.2, acceptable range 2.2–4.2). For any particular IQC sample, the range of INR results should not vary by more than ±0.5 INR units (for example, target 3.2, acceptable limits 2.7–3.7). This should normally be achievable by POC monitors.

In some cases, monitors can be scheduled to prevent test performance until appropriate liquid IQC has been performed.

A written record of IQC results should be maintained to include the INR result, the batch/lot number of test strips employed and the identity of the operator. It is useful to maintain a cumulative record, perhaps as a graph, because this can identify gradual drift in IQC results, which could indicate that the method may be moving out of control; for example, if test strips were deteriorating as a result of inappropriate storage.

Unexpected POC INR results

If an unexpectedly high or unexpectedly low INR result is obtained on a patient's sample, the test should be repeated. Repeat results should normally be within 10% of each other. Any patient INR result of >5.0 should be repeated to confirm that there has not been an analytical error.

Comparing POC INR results with conventional laboratory INR methods

One approach to EQA for POC results is to collect a venous sample at the same time as the POC test and despatch this for analysis in an appropriate hospital laboratory. A protocol for EQA testing should be developed and implemented. EQA may be performed at regular time intervals, or on one sample from each group of patients under investigation, and/or if an unusual INR result on a patient sample is obtained; for example, a markedly high INR. There are difficulties, however, associated with this approach. INR results measured on different systems are not always in agreement with each other. INR results are most reliable for samples within the therapeutic range. Agreement between INR results obtained on different systems may be less good when INRs are above the therapeutic range. It is reasonable to expect good agreement (within 0.5 INR) for samples from stabilised patients on long-term therapy, but where such agreement does not occur, the difficulty may relate to either, or both, of the two method systems being compared. This can complicate interpretation of results obtained when the INR result from a POC device is compared with the INR on a sample from the same patient at the same time measured on a large coagulation analyser in a hospital laboratory. In any case, it should be noted that an INR deviation of up to ±10% has been considered acceptable for clinical purposes. Comparison testing to check the accuracy of the POC device should use samples from patients stable on oral anticoagulants and with no recent changes in diet and no possible interacting drug.

External quality assessment

EQA is available for some POC instruments through the UK National External Quality Assessment Service (UK NEQAS) for Blood Coagulation. Contact details are given at the end of this chapter.

Participation is available to healthcare professionals and is not restricted to the UK. In the scheme, lyophilised plasma samples are provided with all the diluents required, together with a disposable pipette for transfer of diluents to plasma as illustrated in Figure 4.2. No laboratory facilities or equipment are required for analysis. Programmes are currently available for the CoaguChek®, CoaguChek® S, CoaguChek® XS, and CoaguChek® XS Plus devices and for the Hemochron® devices, using either non-citrated or citrated test cuvettes. Samples are specific for each testing device and cannot be compared across programmes. If a centre changes testing device they must ensure that they are in the correct programme for their current device, as failure to do so will make the EQA provided invalid. For all the POC programmes, samples are distributed in four separate surveys per annum. Each centre determines INR, and returns results to the central office for analysis. All results from centres using the same system are grouped together to calculate the median result (middle value when all results are ranked from highest to lowest). If an individual result is within 15% (above or below) of the median for that particular POC monitor, this is considered to be acceptable (within the consensus). If, however, a result is more than 15% higher or more than 15% lower than the median, it is classified as outwith consensus. If this problem occurs repeatedly, then the centre is classified as persistently outwith consensus, and a letter offering support or advice is despatched.

As of 2008, there were five POC monitors employed by ten or more participants in the UK NEQAS (Blood Coagulation scheme) among the 1,500 registered participants.

This is a diverse group, with centres registered in many areas of the healthcare community. Site placement of these devices is shown in Table 4.1, page 26.

For the POC programmes, the percentage coefficient of variance (%CV) is similar to that obtained for INR testing in hospital laboratories, which means that there is a similar degree of imprecision within the methods. The percentage of participating centres

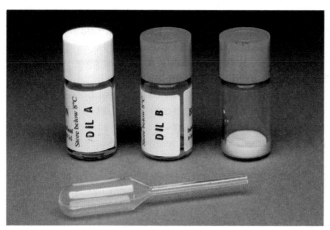

Figure 4.2. Lyophilised plasma and diluents provided by the UK National External Quality Assessment Service scheme for Blood Coagulation for analysis with some POCT monitors. A disposable plastic pipette is provided to transfer diluents and sample

Table 4.1. Location of POC INR devices among participants in the UK NEQAS POC INR program		
Location	Number of participants	% of participants
General practice surgeries and health centres	1,188	77.4%
Hospital laboratories	269	17.5%
Pharmacies	37	2.4%
Hospital outpatient clinics	20	1.3%
Other centres	21	1.4%

whose results are outwith consensus is comparable between the laboratory test programme and the POC test programmes, indicating that performance in the POC test programmes is similar to that in the laboratory test programme. This can be seen in Table 4.2, showing results of sets of eight different samples tested through a) the laboratory programme, b) the CoaguChek® S POC programme and c) the CoaguChek® XS Plus POC programme (note that each programme has a different set of eight samples; therefore, results across programmes cannot be compared). Tables 4.3 and 4.4 (page 27) show the range and % CV of participants' results for samples with median INRs at different levels, as obtained by users of the CoaguChek® S and CoaguChek® XS Plus devices. Overall, these data suggest that EQA is just as necessary for POC monitors as for hospital laboratories.

Results from the UK NEQAS have confirmed that it is possible to identify participants whose results are repeatedly different from those in other centres. In one 12-

Table 4.2. UK NEQAS - INR results with the CoaguChek® instrument					
Laboratory programme		CoaguChek® S		CoaguChek® XS Plus	
INR	% outwith consensus	INR	% outwith consensus	INR	% outwith consensus
3.19	7.1	1.7	6.3	4.5	1.1
1.96	3.8	4.4	15	1.3	2.3
2.1	3.8	3.5	6.2	4.0	0
1.84	5.8	1.1	16.4	3.2	4.0
4.2	12.4	2.8	10.4	2.2	3.1
4.0	9.1	2.7	11.2	4.3	0.4
3.27	6.5	2.6	5.2	3.6	3.1
2.53	5.1	4.2	8.1	2.7	4.2
Mean 2.9	6.7	2.9	9.9	3.2	2.3

Table 4.3. UK NEQAS - INR results with the CoaguChek® S instrument				
Sample	Number of users	Median INR	Range of INRs results received	%CV
1	636	1.7	1.1-5.0	18.7 (9.0)%
2	631	4.4	1.6-8.0	16.3%
3	663	3.5	1.0-8.0	11.8 (8.4)%
4	659	1.1	0.7-3.8	22.9 (11.1)%
5	684	2.8	1.6-8.0	22.4 (14.1)%
6	678	2.7	1.8-8.0	20.1 (13.8)%
7	615	2.6	2.2-8.8	14.0 (9.3)%
8	606	4.2	2.4-8.0	11.9 (10.2)%

%CV = coefficient of variance. Values in parentheses are %CVs with outlying results excluded

month period involving eight test samples, 51 of 96 centres using CoaguChek® or CoaguChek® S and returning results on all samples had all INRs within the acceptable limits. In each survey, approximately 10% of participants had a result outside the acceptable limits, which is similar to hospital laboratory results in the UK NEQAS. Only eight centres had repeated problems, all of which were later able to improve on their performance so that their results were in agreement with other centres. Thus EQA can help to improve agreement in different centres, which is important for proper management of anticoagulant therapy.

Total confidentiality is an important feature of all EQA schemes. Information regarding individual performance in the UK NEQAS is not divulged to anyone other than the nominated personnel.

Table 4.4. UK NEQAS - INR results with the CoaguChek® XS Plus device				
Sample	Number of users	Median INR	Range of INRs	%CV
1	88	4.5	1.40-4.90	8.4 (4.1)
2	89	1.3	1.20-4.80	29.7 (15.0)
3	131	4	3.40-4.40	3.6
4	130	3.2	2.90-4.10	6.2
5	225	2.2	2.10-7.40	25.7 (6.4)
6	227	4.3	2.80-4.70	4.3 (3.6)
7	288	3.6	2.10-5.00	6.7 (5.8)
8	287	2.7	2.40-3.70	7.3 (6.6)

%CV = coefficient of variance. Values in parentheses are %CVs with outlying results excluded

Patients' self-determined INRs

An increasing number of patients determine their own INRs using POC monitors. One of the acceptance criteria before a patient can commence self-testing is the ability to analyse IQC material. Patients should have liquid IQC material available, as described above.

The frequency of IQC testing required to ensure effective anticoagulant control by patient self-testing is not known. In practice, it would be useful to analyse IQC at the following times:

● When introducing a new batch/lot number of test strips
● When introducing use of a newly delivered set of test strips, even if it is the same batch/lot number as previously used
● If there is any doubt about the storage conditions of test strips
● If an unexpected result (higher or lower than expected) is obtained
● At least once every three months.

There are published recommendations (Fitzmaurice *et al* 2005) about IQA and EQA for patients who are self-testing and self-managing, and there are now published data to show that some patients can successfully participate in EQA programmes, such as those described above for healthcare professionals. Based on current evidence, there are three options for external assessment of patients who self-test.

1. A venous sample can be obtained and sent to the hospital laboratory to compare to the POC test INR determined at the same time. This approach has limitations, as discussed above.
2. Patients can be assessed in a clinic that has the same POC monitor and is participating in an accredited EQA programme, such as the UK NEQAS. In this case, the patient should test their INR on their own monitor and also on the monitor in the clinic at the same time. If results are within 0.5 of each other then this would be considered satisfactory.
3. Some patients can successfully test the samples provided through the UK NEQAS and so patients can participate in a programme for INR self-testing, which is similar to the programme for healthcare professionals using these devices.

It seems likely that options 2 or 3 would be most appropriate for patients who determine their own INR with POC monitors.

A NEQAS programme was introduced for patient self-testers who are using the CoaguChek® S device and has been in operation since November 2004. It is required that the patient identifies to the organisers their warfarin provider when they register for the programme. The programme has one test sample per survey, with a survey performed every six months. This is a postal service; the sample is sent to the patient's address and the patient performs the test and sends the result to the UK NEQAS. The data are analysed and a 15% deviation range around the median value is calculated – this is the acceptable range. If the patient is within the acceptable range, they are informed by letter and no further action is required. If, however, their result is outside the range, then a repeat sample is sent for them to retest. If this repeat is within the range, then no further action is taken, but if the repeat test is also outside the acceptable range both the patient and their healthcare provider will receive a letter informing them of this. It is the responsibility of the patient and their healthcare provider to review why the patient's results were outside the range and to resolve this together to

Table 4.5. Results of the UK NEQAS patients self-testers' programme

	S1 n=37	S2 n=41	S3 n=43	S4 n=48	S5 n=146	S6 n=162	S7 n=128	S8 n=115
Median INR for self-testers	1.8	3.1	2.3	3.4	2.9	2.95	2.9	1.7
CV	6%	6%	22%	22%	15%	15%	16%	10%
Range of results	1.6-2.0	2.8-3.4	1.9-5.3	2.6-4.5	2.3-5.4	1.0-8.0	1.6-6.2	1.5-2.6
Number of repeats sent	1	2	3	5	18	22	8	4

ensure that continuing INR monitoring is reliable. As of 2008, eight surveys had taken place, with the results shown in Table 4.5.

The introduction of the CoaguChek® XS device for patient self -testers has further complicated the matter of patients performing quality control, as at present there is no IQC sample for these patients to test

Summary

- Quality assurance (QA) is an overall term used to describe all measures that are taken to ensure the reliability of testing and reporting.
- Internal quality control (IQC) is used to establish whether a particular technique is performing consistently over a period of time in order to ensure that there is day-to-day consistency.
- Many manufacturers of point-of-care (POC) monitors and test strips for international normalised ratio determination have control materials available for the purpose of IQC.
- The frequency of IQC required depends on the number of patient samples analysed.
- If fewer than ten tests are performed within a four-hour period, one IQC should be included.
- If a larger group is tested on the same day, IQC should be performed at the beginning and end of testing.
- External quality assessment (EQA) is used to identify the degree of agreement between one centre's results and those obtained by other centres.
- EQA is available for some POC instruments through the UK National External Quality Assessment Service (UK NEQAS) for Blood Coagulation.

Further reading
Bennett KM, Lader C, Pan C, Zucker ML, Labuca M. Data management and quality assurance compliance for point-of-care coagulation testing. *Clin Chemistry* 2000; **46**: A6.
Fitzmaurice DA, Gardiner C, Kitchen S *et al*. British Society for Haematology Taskforce for Haemostasis and thrombosis. An evidence-based review and guidelines for patient self-testing and management of oral anticoagulation. *Br J Haematol* 2005; **131**: 156–165.
Kitchen S, Walker ID, Woods TAL, Preston FE. Thromboplastin related differences in the determination of

International Normalised Ratio: A cause for concern? *Thromb Haemost* 1994; **72:** 426–429.

Kitchen S, Kitchen DP, Jennings I *et al.* Point of Care INRs: UK NEQAS experience demonstrates necessity for proficiency testing of three different monitors. *Thromb Haemost* 2006; **96:** 590–596.

Murray ET, Jennings I, Kitchen D, Kitchen S, Fitzmaurice DA. Quality assurance for oral anticoagulation self management: a cluster randomized trial. *J Thromb Haemost* 2008; **6:** 464–469.

Murray ET, Kitchen DP, Kitchen S *et al.* Patient self-management of oral anticoagulation and external quality assessment. *Br J Haematol* 2003; **122:** 825–828.

Contact details for UK NEQAS:

UK NEQAS for Blood Coagulation
Rutledge Mews
3 Southbourne Road
Sheffield S10 2QN, UK.
Tel: +44 (0)114 267 3300.
Fax: +44 (0)114 267 3309.
website: www.ukneqasbc.org

Chapter 5

The use of computerised decision support software for anticoagulation management in primary care

Professor DA Fitzmaurice

Learning outcomes

- **The utility of computerised decision support software (CDSS) for anticoagulation management in primary care**
- **The core features of CDSS for processing international normalised ratio (INR) results and managing warfarin therapy**

The traditional model for the management of anticoagulant dosing involved patients attending hospital anticoagulation clinics, where clinicians altered the anticoagulant dose, based upon the patient's international normalised ratio (INR) result. No formal algorithm or mathematical equation was used. GPs in rural areas also used this model. An audit published in 1996 suggested that as few as 50% of UK patients received adequate anticoagulation at any one time and that most patients were not receiving enough anticoagulation. As successful anticoagulation management involves both accurate laboratory determination of INR and accurate dosing – alongside efforts to ensure the standardisation of laboratory techniques and calibration – a variety of algorithms were derived to try to ensure consistent anticoagulant dosing.

Algorithms and mathematical equations for dosing

A variety of simple algorithms have been developed to guide dosing. Some computer systems have simply incorporated these algorithms, while others are based on mathematical equations. Although various attempts have been made to automate the initiation of anticoagulants, most of the systems in current use focus on the maintenance of anticoagulation. In 1984, Wilson and James described an early example of computerised decision support software (CDSS) for managing oral anticoagulation in a hospital setting. They derived rules for adjusting the dose of warfarin based on questionnaires sent to hospital doctors. These rules formed the central logic of their program. An equation was derived from the responses to the questionnaires and the performance achieved using the computer-based equation, compared with that achieved under the manual system. Using 132 patients they demonstrated that the use of the computer system resulted in a fall in the percentage of blood results out of range (from 17.4% to 14.2%), while increasing the mean recall frequency (from 3.91 to 4.84 weeks). Ryan *et al*, in 1989, described an equation that resulted in an increase in the percentage of patients within range from 45.5% to 62.9% over a six-month evaluation. Further algorithms have been proposed by Vadher *et al* and Carter *et al*. Vadher's paper describes an algorithm that uses Bayesian mathematics and pharmacokinetic and pharmacodynamic modelling.

A comparison of various algorithms

There have been several papers describing new techniques for determining a patient's new warfarin dose based upon their INR. These papers often present a comparison with existing manual systems, but there have been very few studies comparing the performance of various equations with each other. However, one study conducted by Poller *et al* in 1993 is noteworthy, as it compares the effectiveness of three computer systems with the customary dosing method. The three equations compared were:
- The Hillingdon system – based upon the algorithm of Wilson and James
- The Charles system – a system used in the Department of Haematology at St Thomas' Hospital in London
- The Coventry program – based upon the algorithm described by Ryan.

Patients were randomised for dosing using one of the four methods. After an initial assessment, use of the Hillingdon system was suspended because of an increased need to amend the dosage and interval suggestions compared with the other systems. Only 12 patients (43 dosings) were managed on this system before suspension, so a statistical comparison with the other systems could not be made. A total of 64 patients (234 dosings) were managed using customary dosing, 57 patients (170 dosings) using the Charles system, and 53 patients (128 dosings) using the Coventry program. The results showed that INR values were within target range on 50.4% of visits for the manual system, 56.5% for the Charles system and 53.1% for the Coventry program. There was no statistically significant difference in the control achieved by these methods. Therefore, the control achieved with these systems is very close to that obtained by experienced medical staff.

Poller also led the largest study in this area, which compared two software systems with manual dosing in a pan-European study of over 13,000 patients and nearly 400,000 INR tests. This study concluded that CDSS was safe and effective in comparison with experienced medical staff dosage at the centres with established interest in anticoagulation. They also claimed that there was significant prevention of clinical events in patients with deep vein thrombosis and pulmonary embolism. This study underpins guidelines for use of CDSS in anticoagulation dosage prepared by the International Society on Thrombosis and Haemostasis.

A systematic review by Fitzmaurice *et al* of CDSS used for oral anticoagulation management identified seven papers describing four different systems. Although this

review noted the paucity of good quality research in the field of CDSS for oral anticoagulation, the above comparison by Poller *et al* scored a maximum score for methodology. This score (Table 5.1) was derived from a point for each of the following:
● Independent blind comparison
● Appropriate sample composition
● Reference standard performed on all patients
● Sufficient description of method to permit replication.

Core CDSS functions

The algorithm used by any system forms the heart of CDSS for oral anticoagulation and enables dosing. A variety of other facilities are often provided by the currently available systems and an examination of these facilities may illustrate additional aspects to consider.

Consultations

The consultation module is used at each patient attendance, with the remaining functions used infrequently to support the consultations. Patients attending for dosing may have a point-of-care test to determine the current INR value, or may have a result from a hospital laboratory. In most of the available systems, the software will cycle through a series of reminders before allowing a consultation. These include notifying the user if the expected date for discontinuing warfarin has been exceeded; reminding the user to ask about adverse events if any were recorded for the current patient on their last visit; and advising of any drug interactions based on the patient's list of medications. Patients are identified on the system and the INR is entered onto the consultation screen. The CDSS then uses its programmed algorithm to determine a new warfarin dose for the patient.

Table 5.1. A systematic review of computerised decision support software		
System	**Paper**	**Methodology score (0-4)**
Hillingdon	Kubie *et al*, 1989	0
Hillingdon	Wyld *et al*, 1988	1
Hillingdon	Wilson and James, 1984	2
PARMA	Mariani *et al*, 1990	1
Coventry	Ryan *et al*, 1989	2
Virginia	Carter *et al*, 1988	1
Hillingdon, Coventry, Charles	Poller *et al*, 1993	4

The CDSS also generates a suggested recall date based upon consensus opinion published in the guidelines from the British Society for Haematology. However, it should be possible to override these recommendations. This is important, as the algorithms used by all the currently available systems take into account relatively few patient parameters when calculating new doses. Clinicians usually consider a variety of additional patient characteristics and circumstances in determining dose changes; for example, poor adherence. These systems merely recommend doses for consideration by the clinician. In many of the available systems, the consultation screen is also used to access details of all the previous consultations, to optionally book the patient into an appointments calendar, to enter details of any medication used by the patient which may interact with warfarin, and to enter any adverse events.

Audit

One of the most important functions of anticoagulation CDSS is audit. Although numerous patient variables can be audited in many different ways (as outlined in Chapter 6), anticoagulation systems must provide information that can be used in primary care to enhance patient care – either by facilitating the management of patients in the clinics, or by allowing comparisons with current anticoagulation literature. Many of these systems will perform an adverse event audit and allow searches for patients who have missed anticoagulation appointments. Some will allow mail-merged letters to be sent to defaulters. The key statistics that primary care anticoagulation systems need to be able to generate include:
● Point prevalence
● Percentage of time spent within range
● Percentage of visits in range
● Review frequency.
   Some systems will also provide a number of other useful facilities such as graphs and printed reports.

Other facilities

Apart from consultation and audit facilities, the systems provide a plethora of additional facilities to aid in the primary care management of oral anticoagulation. These include the ability to back up and restore database files and add data for previous visits, as well as allowing passwords to be changed, amendments to target INRs in light of new guidelines, importing of data from practice systems and the management of clinics.

Comparing systems

A variety of anticoagulation systems are currently in use. Each system has its advantages and disadvantages. When embarking on establishing a new primary care anticoagulation service using CDSS, consideration of a series of questions may be helpful in trying to differentiate the various available systems, such as the following.
● Who is the intended user of this system? Some software has been written for secondary care services and may contain facilities which are not useful in primary care.

- What platform does the software run on? Most modern software runs on a Microsoft Windows® operating system, but should also be compatible with other operating systems.
- Which equation is being used for dosing? Ensure you have investigated the literature demonstrating the efficacy of the equation used by your chosen system.
- Are any useful audit features provided?
- What additional facilities are provided to assist primary care anticoagulation clinics?
- Is the software user-friendly and well supported?
- Is the software cost-effective? Anticoagulation systems vary from £50 to over £5,000. Some companies now offer training as part of their package.
- Does the software integrate with clinical systems?
- Can the software be accessed remotely?

The future for CDSS in primary care anticoagulation

An evolutionary process has seen the metamorphosis of a traditional manual system for managing oral anticoagulation, largely in the secondary care sector, to a more effective, reproducible and auditable patient-centred activity that is feasible in primary care. As with all evolutionary processes, there is scope for further enhancements. The comparability of current equations with expert manual management has been documented. These equations can be further enhanced to produce an even greater proportion of time spent within range and thus further minimise the potential for significant adverse events.

With the greater co-operation seen over the last decade among GP clinical system providers, the key hurdle of data transfer between clinical systems and anticoagulation CDSS is likely to be overcome. This will obviate the need for entering clinical information into two computer systems. With the developments in internet technologies, anticoagulation systems are likely to progress towards internet solutions rather than the current stand-alone applications. An obvious progression in this evolutionary process is in enabling selected patients to manage their own anticoagulation requirements and thereby use CDSS at home. Other technological advances will include use of mobile phones and wireless technology, both for transfer of patient data and for patient alerts.

Finally, the paucity of input variables used by current algorithms and equations may demand the utilisation of artificial intelligence technologies to encapsulate more input variables, as it becomes clearer which additional parameters influence the determination of a recommended warfarin dose and recall interval. All four of these future enhancements to the primary care management of anticoagulation are currently being developed at leading centres.

Summary

- The traditional model of anticoagulant dosing has involved hospital clinicians altering the anticoagulant dose based upon the patient's international normalised ratio (INR) result using no formal algorithm or mathematical equation.

- A variety of simple algorithms have been developed to guide dosing and some computer systems have simply incorporated these algorithms, while others are based upon mathematical equations.
- A program with an algorithm that uses Bayesian mathematics and pharmacokinetic and pharmacodynamic modelling has been described.
- The algorithm used by any system forms the heart of computerised decision support software (CDSS) for oral anticoagulation and enables dosing.
- A variety of other facilities are often provided by the available systems including:
  - **Consultation:** the programmed algorithm is used to determine a new warfarin dose for the patient and to generate a suggested recall date based upon consensus opinion published in the guidelines from the British Society for Haematology
  - **Audit:** anticoagulation systems need to generate statistics that include point prevalence, percentage of time spent within range, percentage of visits in range and review frequency
  - **Other facilities:** the ability to back up and restore database files, add data for previous visits, allow amendments to target INR, import data from practice systems, and manage clinics.
- A variety of anticoagulation systems are currently in use and each system has advantages and disadvantages.
- Anticoagulation CDSS varies in cost from £50 to over £5,000.
- With the development of internet technologies, anticoagulant systems will move towards internet solutions rather than the current stand-alone applications.

Further reading
Rose PE. Audit of anticoagulant therapy. *J Clin Pathol* 1996; **49:** 5–9.
Wilson R, James AH. Computer assisted management of warfarin treatment. *BMJ* 1984; **289:** 422–424.
Ryan PJ, Gilbert M, Rose PE. Computer control of anticoagulant control for therapeutic management. *BMJ* 1989; **299:** 1207–1209.
Kubie A, James AH, Timms J, Brit RP. Experience with a computer-assisted anticoagulant clinic. *Clin Lab Haematol* 1989; **11:** 385–391.
Vadher BD, Patterson DLH, Leaning M. Evaluation of a decision support system for initiation and control of oral anticoagulation in a randomised trial. *BMJ* 1997; **314:** 1252–1256.
Carter BL, Barr W, Rock W, Taylor JW. Warfarin dosage predictions assisted by the analog computer. *Ther Drug Monit* 1988; **10:** 69–73.
Poller L, Wright D, Rowlands J. Prospective comparative study of computer programs used for management of warfarin. *J Clin Pathol* 1993; **46:** 299–303.
Poller L, Keown M, Ibrahim S *et al.* An international multicenter randomized study of computer-assisted oral anticoagulant dosage vs. medical staff dosage. *J Thromb Haemost* 2008; **6:** 935–943.
Fitzmaurice DA, Hobbs FDR, Delaney BC, Wilson S, McManus R. Review of computerized decision support systems for oral anticoagulation management. *Br J Haematol* 1998; **102:** 907–909.
Wyld PJ, West D, Wilson TH. Computer dosing in anticoagulant clinics – the way forward? *Clin Lab Haematol* 1988; **10:** 235–236.
Mariani G, Maotti C, Dettori AG. A computerized regulation of dosage in oral anticoagulant therapy. *Res Clin Lab* 1990; **20:** 119–125.
Blann A, Hewitt J, Siddiqui F, Bareford D. Racial background is a determinant of average warfarin dose required to maintain the INR between 2.0 and 3.0. *Br J Haematol* 1999; **107:** 207–209.
British Committee for Standards in Haematology (BCSH). Guidelines on oral anticoagulation: third edition. *Br J Haematol* 1998; **101:** 374–387.
Vadher BD, Patterson DLH, Leaning M. Prediction of INR and maintenance dose during initiation of warfarin therapy using a Bayesian pharmacokinetic/pharmacodynamic model. *Br J Haematol* 1996; **93**(Suppl 1): 30.

System software manufacturer contact details:

BAP-PC Department of Primary Care and General Practice, The University of Birmingham, Birmingham B15 2TT

DAWN 4S Information Systems, 4 The Square, Milnthorpe, Cumbria LA7 7QJ

EIDER Eider Computers Limited, 11 Beaumont Gate, Radlett, Herts WD7 7AR

INRstar Sullivan Cuff Software Limited, 1 Wheal Agar, Tolvaddon Energy Park, Camborne, Cornwall TR14 0HX

RAT Formulae Software, The Medical Centre, George Avenue, Ballyclare, Northern Ireland BT39 9HL

Chapter 6

Audit parameters for the assessment of anticoagulation clinics

Dr P Kesteven

Learning outcomes

● **The importance of clinical audit**
● **The different parameters for measuring international normalised ratio (INR) control**
● **Additional measurable parameters to ensure total quality care with an anticoagulant clinic**

Oral anticoagulants have a narrow therapeutic window, requiring regular titration of dose against anticoagulant effect as determined by the international normalised ratio (INR). Deviation from the target range, in either direction, is associated with a sharp increase in adverse events (Figure 6.1).

There are many ways of organising anticoagulant clinics – a number of which are described in this book. Considering the large (and growing) number of patients who

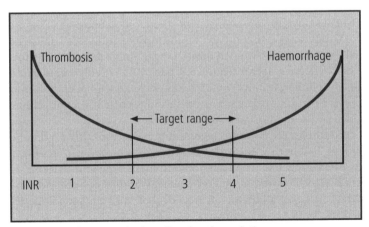

Figure 6.1. Risks versus the benefits of anticoagulation

are receiving oral anticoagulants and the range of facilities available across the country, it seems likely that this variety of clinic models will remain. Despite (perhaps because of) these variations in service delivery, it is vital that the clinics are audited and benchmarks maintained. The purpose of this chapter is to help answer the question: can we be certain that our anticoagulant clinics are doing their job? In other words, are we actually doing what we think we are doing, and how does what we do compare to pre-determined standards or benchmarks?

Each component of the warfarin service should be subjected to regular audit and review, including sample collection and handling, suitable techniques for testing, up-to-date standard operating procedures (SOPs) and appropriate documentation (see Chapter 4). This chapter will cover the audit of laboratory measurements, dosing, patient satisfaction and clinic administration, which incorporates all of the above. Clinical outcomes will also be discussed, although strictly speaking this is not a component of the audit of anticoagulant clinics.

Audit of laboratory measurements

A key consideration is whether or not the INR is being determined both precisely and accurately. This is usually ascertained by the measurement of control samples, which are handled in exactly the same way as routine, clinical samples. There are two types of quality control (QC) material. The first is a sample of blood with a known INR value – internal QC (IQC) – which is tested frequently. In a busy laboratory, this may be with each batch of samples. The series of results obtained should remain within tight limits around the known INR value. Results falling outside these limits will alert the operator to a 'drift' in the standard of equipment or the reagents.

The second type of QC is a sample of unknown INR value, again tested by the same method as routine samples. This material is provided, and the results assessed, by an independent external body. The largest UK body providing external QC for anticoagulation is the UK National External Quality Assessment Service (NEQAS).

Supply of IQC material is usually organised by the local haematology laboratory or, in the case of automated point-of-care (POC) equipment, by the manufacturer. It is recommended that IQC samples be tested at least once for each clinic day, whenever reagents or batches of 'strips' are changed, or whenever an unusual INR result is found. A vital part of this process is that the QC results must be monitored and action taken if the results fall outside predetermined limits. One example demonstrates the influence of a change in a batch of reagents (Figure 6.2, page 40). A highly significant drift in the mean INR for the clinic was noted, which was associated with alterations in mean warfarin doses prescribed. The cause of the drift was identified as a stabilising agent that had been added by the manufacturer of the reagent.

External QC samples are issued at regular intervals – monthly for laboratories and quarterly for POC INR testing. Individual results are compared with results from across the country and segregated according to equipment type and reagents used. In no sense is there a 'right' answer, but merely the reassurance of how one clinic's results compare with every other laboratory. A great deal of work has been undertaken examining external QC for POC coagulometers (see Chapter 4).

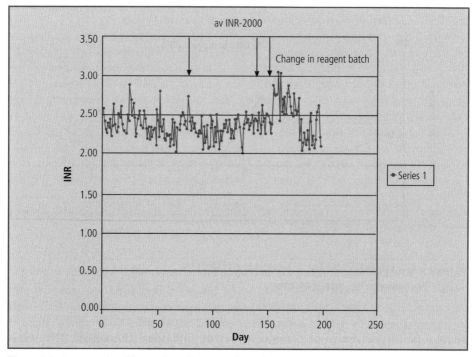

Figure 6.2. An example of internal quality control results

Dosing

Once the INR has been determined correctly, it is important to confirm that the appropriate dose of anticoagulant is being prescribed (Figure 6.3, page 41). Computer-aided systems are now used frequently, and commercially available software has usually been verified in this regard. Nevertheless, systems differ (see Chapter 5) and, regardless of whether a computer is used or not, it is important to verify that a safe and therapeutic INR has been achieved. One endpoint for this is the incidence of adverse events. However, there are two drawbacks to using this as an audit parameter. The first is that serious adverse events are relatively rare and may be extremely difficult to identify. Second, as discussed below, the occurrence of these complications may not necessarily be a reflection of the efficacy of the anticoagulant clinic.

The level of therapeutic control may be expressed in terms of the proportion of all INRs that are within the therapeutic range. Methods of expressing this include:
- Point prevalence – the proportion of patients with therapeutic INRs
- The proportion of tests performed that are within the therapeutic range
- The proportion of time spent by individuals in the therapeutic range.

Point prevalence

This is the most widely reported method and simply calculates the proportion of patients achieving individual therapeutic INRs at a given time. Hospital-based clinics

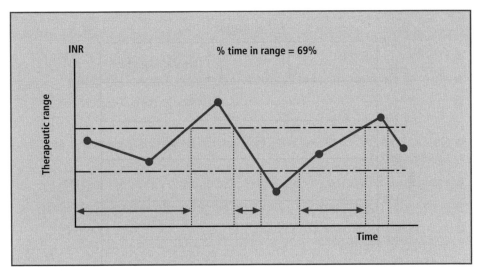

Figure 6.3. A method for calculating the percentage time in range, which is based on assuming a straight line between INR measurements

show a point prevalence of patients achieving individual therapeutic INR levels of 43–55%. This compares with a figure of 54% in general practice clinics using similar methods.

Proportion of tests within range

This method considers a number of INR measurements within the target range expressed as a percentage of the total number of values obtained. It therefore gives a more representative view of the clinic performance as a whole, with more unstable patients contributing a greater proportion of results than patients who are well controlled. Typical clinic results are 50–60% within 0.5 INR units of the target.

Proportion of time spent in range

There has been some disagreement over how best to determine the time spent in range for an individual patient and various formulae have been tested. For instance, a patient with a particular INR value can be assumed to have had that value for the whole period since the previous test; to have had that value for half the time since the test was taken; or to have had a linear change in INR between the two readings. The linear change method is generally accepted as the best in this regard as it recognises that a patient who is below the therapeutic range at the first visit but above at the second must have spent some time within the therapeutic zone. This method of calculating therapeutic control gives values intermediate to the two previously mentioned.

The British Society for Haematology (BSH) has produced guidelines relating to several readily obtainable measures of the dosing efficiency of the clinic (Table 6.1, page 42). With regard to dosing, the recommendations are 50% of INRs within 0.5 INR units

> ## Table 6.1. Standards for audit (British Society for Haematology guidelines)
>
> - Provision of adequate data for safe transfer of anticoagulant follow-up
> - Provision of anticoagulant cards for patients on hospital discharge
> - Patient information: awareness of the need for anticoagulation and possible side-effects of the treatment
> - Hospital notes contain information that the patient is currently taking warfarin
> - The use of heparin/warfarin dosage schedules in a hospital setting
> - Follow-up arrangements for patients failing to attend appointments
> - Achievement of target INR: 50% of INRs within 0.5 INR units, and 80% within 0.75 INR units, of target
>
> NB: Significantly, of these seven criteria only one refers to testing or dosing

and 80% within 0.75 INR units of target. Other simple measures include mean INR with standard deviation for the individual clinic.

Whichever audit parameters of INR dosing are chosen, allowances must be made for interindividual variations in response to oral anticoagulants. For a given target INR (for example, 2.5) a wide range of doses is required; with warfarin this may range from less than 1 mg to more than 20 mg daily. Reasons for this variation include age, size, liver function, diet, compliance, alcohol use and other medications. Even making allowances for these factors, it is clear that patients vary in 'sensitivity' to changes in warfarin dose, for reasons that are not yet well understood. Some have argued that this sensitivity may be due to borderline vitamin K deficiency. Others have shown that variations in cytochrome P450 (a liver enzyme that metabolises warfarin) is associated with lower maintenance dose requirements and an increased risk of haemorrhagic complications on starting anticoagulation. It is important to note that audit parameters of dosing will be influenced by the proportion of 'sensitive' patients attending the clinic (Appendix 6.1, page 45).

Patient satisfaction

Many anticoagulant clinics assess patients' satisfaction with, for example, siting and timing of clinics, or response times for results or advice. This should be a regular feature. The level of patient knowledge, or the effect of patient education at initiation, is more difficult to determine. It has been demonstrated that anticoagulant control will be better and safer in those patients who understand how this medication works and who can anticipate likely adverse interactions. Indeed, recent research has demonstrated that patient information leaflets are generally well understood and have a beneficial effect. Efforts should be made to audit this aspect of the service regularly.

Administration

This may now be the most important element of an anticoagulant service requiring audit. Patients 'lost' to the system – such that they either remain on anticoagulants but fail to have this monitored, or that they have stopped taking anticoagulants when these should continue – are at serious risk of suffering an adverse event. It could be argued that this risk is at least as great as those engendered by failings in testing or dosing elements. Thus, care should be taken to monitor all patients in the system, to chase those failing to attend appointments and, where relevant, to ensure that transfer of patients (and their details) between secondary and primary care is timely and complete. It is also very important to ensure that both target INRs and the duration of anticoagulation are consistent with the diagnosis. Most importantly, no patient should be anticoagulated for longer than necessary. The benchmark for this element of the service should be 100% compliance.

Clinical outcomes

As with any therapy it is extremely important to determine clinical outcomes as the final determinant of its therapeutic value. However, this may represent research , as opposed to audit. Both haemorrhagic and thrombotic complications of oral anticoagulants are closely related to the INR. For instance, the relative risk of serious bleeding doubles with each unit increase in INR. However, looking at the problem the other way around, one series examined all cases of intracranial haemorrhage presenting to a tertiary referral centre over a five-year period, of whom 116 were taking anticoagulants. Two-thirds of this group experienced haemorrhage when the INR was either in or below the therapeutic range, while one-third should not (by accepted guidelines) have been on anticoagulants in the first place. Thus, a patient on warfarin may suffer a significant bleed while the INR is in the therapeutic range. This obviously has clinical significance and may engender debate on patient selection and indications for anticoagulation, but provides little useful information concerning the workings of an anticoagulant clinic itself.

Summary

- Deviation from the target international normalised ratio (INR), in either direction, is associated with a sharp increase in adverse events. Therefore, it is vital that the clinics are audited and benchmarks maintained.
- Components of the warfarin service for regular audit and review are:
  - **Laboratory measurements:** whether the INR is determined precisely and accurately, ascertained by the measurement of control samples, internal quality control and external quality assessment
  - **Dosing:** whether the appropriate dose of anticoagulant is prescribed. It is important to verify that a safe and therapeutic INR has been achieved using point prevalence (the proportion of patients with a therapeutic INR); the proportion of tests performed that are within the therapeutic range; and the proportion of time spent by individuals in the therapeutic range
  - **Patient satisfaction:** regarding the siting and times of clinics; response times for

results or advice and information to determine the level of patient knowledge; or the effect of patient education at initiation
  - **Clinic administration:** care should be taken to monitor all patients within the system, to chase those failing to attend appointments and to ensure that the transfer of all patients between secondary and primary care is timely and complete.
- No patient should receive anticoagulation for longer than necessary.
- It is extremely important to determine clinical outcomes, as with any therapy, as the final determinant of its therapeutic value. However, this may represent research as opposed to audit.
- A patient on warfarin may suffer a significant bleed while the INR is in the therapeutic range, which has clinical significance and may engender debate on patient selection and indications for anticoagulation. However, this provides little useful information concerning the workings of an anticoagulant clinic itself.

Further reading
Ryan PJ, Gilbert M, Rose PE. Computer control of anticoagulant dose for therapeutic management. *BMJ* 1989; **299:** 1207–1209.
Rosendaal F, Cannegieter S, van der Meer F, Briet E. A method to determine the optimal intensity of oral anticoagulant therapy. *Thromb Haemostas* 1993; **69:** 236–239.
Aithal GP, Day CP, Kesteven PJ, Daly AK. Association of polymorphisms in the cytochrome P450 CYP2C9 with warfarin dose requirement and risk of bleeding complications. *Lancet* 1999; **353:** 717–719.
Mattle H, Kohler S, Huber P, Rohner M, Steinsiepe K. Anticoagulation-related intracranial extracerebral haemorrhage. *J Neurol Neurosurg Psych* 1989; **52:** 829–837.
British Committee for Standards in Haematology (BCSH). Guidelines on oral anticoagulation: third edition. *Br J Haematol* 1998; **101:** 374–387.

Appendix 6.1. 'Wobble' factor

We determined the standard deviation (SD) of international normalised ratios (INRs) in 500 patients, based on INRs measured over a six-month period, including only those who had been receiving anticoagulants for at least nine months (that is, excluding those just starting). It may be seen that the degree of 'wobble' (the size of the SD) increased dramatically with the target INR. Furthermore, each target range group demonstrated a long tail of very high SDs. Traditionally, patients with these chronically 'unstable' INR results have been assumed to be poorly compliant – usually with medication but also with diet and alcohol intake. In some cases this is probably true. However, it is apparent that there is a large variation within the population in sensitivity to changes in warfarin dose. This is most apparent in the rate at which the INR falls after stopping medication (for instance, in preparation for surgery).

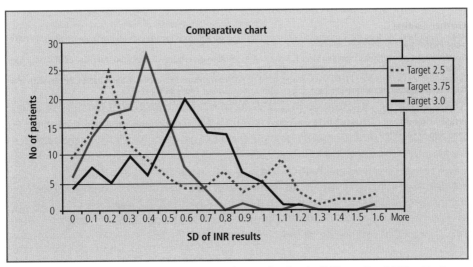

The standard deviation (SD) of the international normalised ratio (INR) results of 500 patients over six months, indicating that the degree of 'wobble' increases with the target INR

Appendix 6.2. Safety indicators for anticoagulant services

The National Patient Safety Agency and the British Committee for Standards in Haematology have identified safety indicators for inpatient and ambulatory anticoagulant services. Indicators have been developed for starting and maintaining anticoagulant therapy. Monitoring these indicators will help to identify risks and promote the appropriate action to minimise them.

Safety indicators for patients starting oral anticoagulant treatment

1 Percentage of patients following loading protocol.
2 Percentage of patients developing international normalised ratio (INR) >5.0.
3 Percentage of patients in therapeutic range at discharge.
4 Percentage (incidence) of patients suffering a major bleed in first month of therapy,

and percentage suffering major bleed with INR above therapeutic range.

5 Percentage of new referrals to anticoagulant service (hospital or community-based) with incomplete information; for example, diagnosis, target INR, stop date for antico-agulant therapy, dose of warfarin on discharge and list of other drugs on discharge.

6 Percentage of patients that were not issued with patient-held information and writ-ten dosage instructions at start of therapy.

7 Percentage of patients that were discharged from hospital without an appointment for the next INR measurement or for consultation with appropriate healthcare profes-sional to review and discuss treatment plan, benefits, risks and patient education.

8 Percentage of patients with subtherapeutic INR when heparin stopped.

Safety indicators for patients established on oral anticoagulant treatment

1 Proportion of patient-time in range (if this is not measurable because of inadequate decision support software then secondary measure of percentage of INRs in range should be used).

2 Percentage of INRs >5.0.

3 Percentage of INRs >8.0.

4 Percentage of INRs >1.0 INR unit below target (for example, percentage of INRs <1.5 for patients with target INR of 2.5).

5 Percentage of patients suffering adverse outcomes, categorised by type, such as a major bleed.

6 Percentage of patients lost to follow-up (and risk assessment of process management for identifying patients lost to follow-up).

7 Percentage of patients with unknown diagnosis, target INR or stop date.

8 Percentage of patients with inappropriate target INR for diagnosis, high and low.

9 Percentage of patients without written patient education information.

10 Percentage of patients without appropriate clinical information; for example, diag-nosis, target INR, last dosing record.

Chapter 7

Anticoagulation management in primary care

Dr ET Murray

Professor DA Fitzmaurice

Learning outcome

- **How primary care can undertake oral anticoagulation management using point-of-care testing for international normalised ratio (INR) measurement and computerised decision support software for management of results**

Effective management of warfarin requires the following: phlebotomy to measure the international normalised ratio (INR); interpretation of the result; advice on the warfarin dosage; and management of the complications of therapy.

Historically in the UK, anticoagulation management has been undertaken mostly within hospital outpatient clinics under the care of haematology laboratories and consultant haematologists. However, in recent years there has been a degree of movement to models of care outside hospital services, including management by the patient.

There is now increasing evidence that specialised clinics within primary care using point-of-care (POC) devices to measure the INR are able to achieve high standards of complete anticoagulation management with little input from the service laboratory. Specialised clinics have since been developed in the USA and have endorsed findings of minimised risks when anticoagulation is monitored within these clinics.

Planning a primary care service

With the introduction of practice-based commissioning (following 2004 Department of Health [DH] guidance), the government aims to devolve appropriate services to a primary care setting in order to develop more locally provided services and to reduce the number of outpatient referrals into secondary care. The delivery of primary care anticoagulation monitoring would provide seamless care between the primary/secondary care interface, in that appropriate patients would receive continuing primary care with access to secondary care as necessary. The success of implementing primary care anticoagulation services can be evaluated by evidence of reduction in secondary care activity, patient waiting times, improved access to services and improved patient choice. Evidence shows that GPs or other healthcare professionals, such as practice nurses, with or without computerised decision support software (CDSS), are able to achieve high standards of anticoagulation care.

Anticoagulation monitoring is a national enhanced service (NES) that can be offered by GP practices that have adequate experience, training and competence in this field. The terms for delivery of this type of service have been set out by the British Medical Association (BMA) (http://www.bma.org.uk).

Four levels of service are recognised and remuneration for the service is geared accordingly – offering up to £127.86 for a full level 4 service, as outlined below:

- Level 1 – Laboratory outreach sampling, test and dose
- Level 2 – Health authority, trust or other externally funded phlebotomist or pharmacist, practice sample, laboratory test, practice dosing
- Level 3 – Practice-funded phlebotomist or pharmacist, practice sample, laboratory test, practice dosing
- Level 4 – Practice-funded phlebotomist or pharmacist, practice sample, practice test, practice dosing.

In addition to the above fees, if a member of the practice staff undertakes a domiciliary visit to perform a blood test, an extra £3–5 is awarded.

Other remuneration for this service is through Quality and Outcomes Framework indicators for atrial fibrillation (AF), which include points for producing a register of AF patients, the number with confirmed diagnosis and the number treated with anticoagulant therapy.

Levels 1 and 2

Phlebotomy only, with dosing decisions made by a hospital department

This is a widespread model, whereby patients receive dosing information through the post or by telephone. This model retains the expertise and quality assurance (QA) of the laboratory process while at the same time decentralising at a minimal cost to primary care. Patients can attend their GP's surgery and a venous blood sample is then sent to the central laboratory.

The INR is determined and information on dosage and the next appointment is sent to the patient. There are no clinically significant changes in the INR when analysis is delayed for up to three days and the quality control with POC sampling is at least equal to that within a hospital-based setting. This process requires access to phlebotomy in general practice, while the cost of testing and dosing remains with the central laboratory.

Level 3

Phlebotomy plus dosing within the practice, analysis of INR made by a hospital laboratory

General practices with limited access to hospital clinics are more likely to undertake the level of care involving dosing advice. GPs who do not have access to CDSS appear to have much the same difficulty as hospital clinics in their efforts to achieve optimum INR control, with only approximately 50% of patients achieving therapeutic INRs.

Level 4

Complete anticoagulation service in the community: the Birmingham model

The Birmingham model of care comprises POC for INR estimation and CDSS for recommendation of dosage and recall, within a practice nurse-led clinic. Patients attending clinics were assessed for 12 months and compared to control patients attending hospital clinics during the same period. INR therapeutic range, analysed as point prevalence, proportion of tests in range and proportion of time in range, all compared favourably to the hospital control patients. The number of serious adverse events in the practice population was also reduced.

The CDSS aided in the interpretation of results, although it could be overridden if the suggestion made was not clinically indicated. It was essential to ensure that formal training and QA procedures for the POC were in existence at the initial stages of the clinic development, in order to offer an effective and reliable service. This model of care gives an immediately available result which, in turn, offers the patient a complete model of care.

The pharmacist model

Another primary care model that has undergone limited evaluation is a pharmacist-managed anticoagulant clinic. This model again uses POC for INR estimation, and dosing is undertaken by an unaided practitioner. This study demonstrated 90% of patients achieving therapeutic INRs (±10%), with a cost to the practice of less than £35 per attendance. Although no formal details of patient satisfaction evaluation were stated, it was claimed that patients preferred surgery management and welcomed reduced waiting times and travelling costs. The study also claimed improved patient understanding, which may have been an aid to compliance. Further pharmacist-managed clinics are currently being evaluated.

Other models

Biomedical and clinical scientists are now moving from the traditional role within the laboratory setting to successfully managing anticoagulation within secondary care and satellite primary clinics throughout the UK. Patients are also managing their own warfarin using POC testing and a simple dosage chart. This model is discussed in Chapter 10.

Service outline

Having demonstrated that a decentralised community-based system is workable, one then has to answer the concerns expressed about QA and monitoring of therapy.

Funding for the enhanced service, at whatever level, is dependent on certain conditions. Therapy should be initiated normally in secondary care for specified lengths of time and properly controlled maintenance of patients should be practised. The service should be convenient to the patient and treatment need should be continually reviewed. Therapy should be discontinued when appropriate.

To ensure the above service, funding will be allocated for the development and maintenance of a patient register; call and recall; professional links; referral policies; education and newly diagnosed patients; individual management plans; clinical procedures; record-keeping and audit; training and review.

The document emphasises that anyone involved in the enhanced service of anticoagulation management needs to be professionally qualified, in that they have satisfactory training and competences. Healthcare professionals involved in anticoagulation management should be familiar with the updated British Committee for Standards in Haematology (BCSH) guidelines, the National Institute for Health and Clinical Excellence (NICE) guidelines for atrial fibrillation, the National Service Framework (NSF) for Coronary Heart Disease and the 2007 National Patient Safety Agency (NPSA) report.

In 2006, the NPSA undertook a risk assessment of anticoagulant use and produced five overarching strategies for improving safety of delivery:
- Rationalise product ranges and use products with safer designs
- Provide patients with better information and improve communication
- Ensure up-to-date and clearly written policies and procedures – which are followed
- Provide training to ensure defined work competences to safely use medicine
- Produce annual medicines management audits and reports.

The NPSA risk assessment in 2006 found 120 recorded deaths and 480 serious harms from anticoagulant use and that anticoagulants were the second therapeutic group (after opiates) causing the most deaths and severe harm.

As a result, a report was produced outlining implementation of strategies for safer delivery, comprising risk assessment tools (audit parameters); updated patient-held information booklets (yellow books) to ensure patients have adequate information; posters for dental surgeries recommending INR levels for treatment; clinical guidelines and protocols – including those for medicines interacting with warfarin, daily dosing of warfarin, recommendation for the use of computerised decision support software (CDSS), and prescribing and dispensing warfarin; and recommendations for work competences.

To aid evaluation of the service, it produced patient safety indicators, audit protocols and audit collection forms. Action deadlines were set for the DH Safety Alert Broadcast System (SABS) for an action plan to be agreed and actions started by July 2007 and a deadline for all actions to be implemented by 31 March 2008. The Central Alerting System replaced SABS in September 2008 (see https://www.cas.dh.gov.uk).

The following protocol has been developed to incorporate all of the above factors and can be adapted at a local level to suit the requirements of an individual practice. It outlines a typical anticoagulation management protocol and covers all elements that practices in either a primary or secondary care setting would need to consider in developing their own service.

An exemplar protocol for an oral anticoagulation clinic using POC systems and CDSS

Aim

The aim of the service is to offer standardised and clinically effective anticoagulation management for patients receiving anticoagulation therapy.

Objectives

- To receive, manage and ensure appropriate referral of patients who require anticoagulation therapy and are registered in the practice
- To ensure all patients have a treatment plan reviewed on a regular basis (annually)
- To identify patients with specific needs; for example: poor compliance, unstable INR control or frequent non-attenders for review by designated clinician
- To educate new and review patients in understanding their treatment, in terms of their condition requiring warfarin, target range for INR, the effects of over- and under-anticoagulation, diet, lifestyle and drug interactions
- To advise on an anticoagulant regimen before surgery or dental care (BCSH guidelines)
- To provide optimum care in terms of:
  1. INR control; for example, 60–70% of individual patients' INR tests in range at any given time
  2. Identifying and managing clinical events related to warfarin therapy
  3. Considering the impact of patient choice (patient satisfaction questionnaire annually; for example, accessibility, waiting time, and continuity of care)
- To evaluate the quality of care given through regular audit process, effecting change when required to achieve planned goals
- To ensure relevant, complete and accurate documentation of the clinic process
- To undertake an annual review and update of the protocol.

Specific objectives for primary care only

- To initiate and manage warfarin therapy for patients with AF in the general practice clinic.

Capacity

All patients receiving warfarin therapy are referred to the clinic.

Exceptions

- Patients under 16 years of age
- Following discussion with a specialist, patients with complex pathologies, such as atypical systemic emboli, anything not listed under routine indications for warfarin
- Domiciliary patients. Although practices will need to make a decision regarding patients requiring home visiting, they are the group that would most benefit from primary care services
- Patients choosing to continue with hospital/primary care.

Exclusions (nurse-led in acute care)
- Patients with complex pathologies whose management is beyond the competence of the nurse.

Indications for warfarin use and target INR

The indications and targets are taken from British Society for Haematology guidelines. Other targets will be acceptable for named patients after discussion with a designated clinician.

Target INR 2.5
Pulmonary embolus
Proximal deep vein thrombosis
Calf vein thrombosis
Recurrence of venous thromboembolism
Non-rheumatic AF
AF with other causes
Mural thrombus
Cardiomyopathy
Symptomatic inherited thrombophilia
Antiphospholipid syndrome
Bioprosthetic valve if anticoagulated
Arterial grafts if anticoagulated
Mechanical prosthetic aortic valve (or 3.0)
Cardioversion (or 3.0)

Target INR 3.5
Recurrence of venous thromboembolism while on warfarin therapy
Mechanical prosthetic valve (or 3.0)

Not indicated
Ischaemic stroke without AF
Retinal vein occlusion
Peripheral arterial thrombosis and grafts
Coronary artery thrombosis
Coronary artery graft thrombosis
Coronary angioplasty and stents

Risk management

Assess risk to both the patient and the healthcare professional. Implement risk reduction strategies incorporated into the clinic management; for example, patient selection and development of clinic protocol.

Management of clinic

- Allocate protected time per week for clinic but availability for emergency services other days
- Inform hospital/primary care clinics currently managing patient of new clinic
- Train a nurse in anticoagulation management to manage the clinic with support from a designated clinician
- Estimate the INR using a POC device
- Interpret the INR result with the assistance of CDSS
- Perform internal quality control at the start of each clinic and after every 20 INR tests using material supplied by the manufacturer
- Perform external quality control every three months using samples from an external quality assessment scheme, such as the Common External Quality Assessment System (CEQAS) or UK National External Quality Assessment Service (NEQAS)
- Adhere to health and safety procedures recommended by laboratory staff to protect both the patient and clinical staff at all times.

Identify key personnel

Establish effective routes of communication between some of the following:
- Haematologist/anticoagulant nurse specialist (named)
- Lead GP (named)
- Lead practice nurse (named)
- Laboratory contact (named)
- Anticoagulant clinic contact (named)
- Pharmacist
- ICT personnel
- Administrator.

Training

The clinic will be managed by trained staff (designated users). Personnel responsible for the clinic are aware of professional accountability and undertake the clinic management only if they feel competent to do so. Accredited courses are available. Personnel managing the clinic will also be aware of continued professional development and attend regular updates on anticoagulation management. A patient group direction may be used if nurse prescribing is to be initiated. If supplementary prescribing by nurses and pharmacists is to be undertaken their names must be annotated on their professional registers to indicate successful completion of recognised prescribing training. Training should include:
- An introduction to oral anticoagulation therapy, an understanding of the test to be performed, the INR and how it is derived
- An understanding of a specific POC device for deriving INR, setting up and using it
- The target INR, how it relates to diagnosis, action if results are outside limits
- Recording of results and QA materials
- Health and safety – disposal of sharps, Control of Substances Hazardous to Health (COSHH) regulations.

Standard operating procedures will be needed when using POC devices (see Appendix 7.1, page 59).

Identification and referral of patients

Referrals from other clinics or specialists

For primary care, the practice computer database will identify most patients. In addition, patients can be identified from warfarin prescriptions. Regular computer searches (every three months) will check for new patients to the practice receiving warfarin.

Hospital/primary care anticoagulant clinics will need to be informed of all patients attending other clinics. A letter should be sent to the hospital/primary care clinic to inform them if another clinic is going to take over the anticoagulation monitoring. A referral letter should include clinical indication, recommended period on warfarin and target INR. An example referral form is shown in Appendix 7.2, page 61.

Telephone referrals cannot be accepted unless under exceptional circumstances.

All patients will remain the responsibility of the referring centre until the patient is seen in the clinic.

For patients moving to a new practice, hospital clinics will be informed if patients need to be referred back to the hospital clinic. The same referral form will be used attached to a referral letter with a copy to the patient and new GP, if known.

Primary care

Patients can attend the practice clinic once their INR has been within therapeutic range on two occasions. At this point, the hospital clinic can discharge the patient into GP care if appropriate arrangements have been made. (Acute thromboses and other conditions may be referred on discharge.)

Clinic procedure

- Prepare POC device and complete internal quality control procedure. Document control result, batch numbers, and so forth
- Counsel patient regarding clinic process and check for:
  - Bleeding or thrombotic incidences
  - Tablet compliance and change of medication
  - Lifestyle changes (for example, alcohol binges)
- Perform blood test using capillary blood. Venous samples can be taken at a patient's request or for capillary results greater than POC upper limits
- Perform INR test using POC device and enter results into the CDSS
- Follow suggestions given by computer for dosing and recall dates unless clinically inappropriate (for example, patient known to be non-compliant with therapy)
- Complete patient record card and give to patient with verbal instruction regarding dosage and recall
- Record INR, warfarin dosage and recall date in patient's notes and practice computer
- Back up computer software at the end of each clinic.

Annual review

- Assess condition requiring warfarin – risk/benefit – at annual specialist or clinician follow-up; check recommended period of time on warfarin
- Assess whether warfarin therapy is still appropriate
- Assess patient satisfaction using a simple questionnaire.

New patients

- Review treatment plans of all new patients, ensure all patient details are entered and correct in both yellow record book and referral letter and patient is given information sheets and record book
- Ensure that patient has correct target range, duration of treatment for condition requiring warfarin. If not, referring clinician should be consulted
- Educate about warfarin treatment, target range, effects of over- and under-anticoagulation, diet, lifestyle and drug interactions
- Explain the clinic system with regard to blood testing, dosing and next test date.

Clinical guidelines for initiation of warfarin

Patients having warfarin initiated for AF in the community should have a baseline INR performed. Warfarin should only be initiated if the baseline INR is less than 1.3. Any patient with a baseline INR of 1.3 or above should be screened for underlying conditions. Check full blood counts, liver function tests and clotting screen. The initiation dose for patients commencing warfarin for AF in the community should be 1–3 mg daily. Check INR after one week and then weekly until INR is within therapeutic range and then dose according to result using CDSS.

Clinical guidelines for over-anticoagulation

If INR greater than 5.0 on POCT (see also Table 7.1, page 56):
- Assess for clinical signs of bleeding and consider administration of vitamin K (in practice clinic or refer to hospital A&E)
- If no bleeding, follow CDSS guidelines for suspension of treatment
- If bleeding, refer to GP/hospital
- If INR greater than 8.0, refer to hospital for vitamin K administration (IV preparation given orally or IV)
- Check INR the next day.

Definition of serious and non-serious adverse events

Serious adverse event

- Bleeding: if admitted to hospital or if surgery was required to stop bleeding and if bleeding led to reduction of Hb of 2 g/dl or more and/or requiring blood transfusion

Table 7.1. BSH guidelines for INR greater than 5.0	
INR>3.0 and <6.0 (Target 2.5) **INR>4.0 and <6.0** (Target 3.5)	Reduce or stop warfarin; restart when INR <5.0
INR>6.0 and <8.0 No bleeding or minor bleeding	Stop warfarin; restart when INR <5.0
INR >8.0 No bleeding or minor bleeding	Stop warfarin; restart when INR <5.0 If other risk factors for bleeding, give 0.5-2.5 mg of vitamin K (oral)
Major bleeding	Stop warfarin; admit to hospital for urgent reversal (prothrombin complex concentrate/FFP [fresh frozen plasma]) and IV vitamin K 5-10 mg.

- Thrombotic: transient ischaemic attack (with observed neurological deficit) or stroke, recurrent deep vein thrombosis and pulmonary embolism, systemic embolism.

Non-serious
- All cases of bleeding with no associated costs or medical consequences; for example, bruising, small epistaxis, microscopic haematuria.

Advice to patient having dental treatment

Patients are advised to continue with warfarin therapy when attending for dental treatment. However, they will need to check their INR the day before the appointment to ensure the INR is below 4.0.

Preoperative management of warfarin

- If major surgery – stop warfarin four days before surgery; heparin introduced preoperatively in hospital.
- If minor surgery – reduce INR to approximately 2.0 on day of surgery (liaise with hospital to discuss warfarin dosage on discharge).

Guidelines for discontinuing warfarin

To discontinue warfarin at treatment completion, obtain written confirmation from clinician that commenced warfarin therapy. The end date of treatment should be clarified on the original referral form.

Administrative tasks

- Contact non-attendees to the clinic with a letter/telephone call and a new appointment.
- Perform a weekly computer search for non-attendees to warfarin clinic.
- Forward anticoagulant therapy cards of patients who have moved away to designated GP or re-refer to hospital anticoagulant clinic if necessary.
- Perform a backup of software at the end of each clinic.

Audit (safety indicators)

To be performed at least annually, reviewed and changes made where needed.
- INR results in terms of percentage time in range and point prevalence
- Mean INR and mean warfarin dose
- IQC and EQA results
- Adverse events in terms of major and minor events – defined according to previously accepted criteria described above
- Patient satisfaction
- Numbers attending the clinics
- Attendance rate and waiting time
See NPSA report for further parameters.

This protocol has been developed on behalf of the PCT by:

                                    Signed   Date

Lead Doctor

Lead Pharmacist

Lead Nurse

Head of Primary Care

Quality Control

Consultation with:

Summary

- Managing warfarin effectively requires phlebotomy to measure the international normalised ratio (INR); interpretation of the result; advice on the warfarin dosage and management of the complications of therapy.
- Anticoagulation management has been identified in the 2006 GMS contract as one of the services requiring additional funding as a national enhanced service.
- Evidence shows that primary care professionals, with or without computerised decision support software (CDSS), are able to achieve high standards of anticoagulation care.
- The Birmingham model of care comprises point-of-care for INR estimation and CDSS for recommendation of dosage and recall, within a practice nurse-led clinic.
- The aim of the primary care-based clinic is to offer standardised and clinically effective anticoagulation management to primary care patients receiving warfarin therapy.
- The NPSA has produced a number of safety indicators for safe management of oral anticoagulation.

Further reading
Ansell J. Anticoagulation Management as a Risk Factor for Adverse Events: Grounds for Improvement. *J Thromb Thrombolysis* 1998; **5**(Suppl 1): 13–18.
Rose PE. Audit of anticoagulation therapy. *J Clin Pathol* 1996; **49:** 5–9.
Fitzmaurice DA, Hobbs FDR, Murray ET, Bradley C, Holder R. Evaluation of computerized decision support for oral anticoagulation management based in primary care. *Br J Gen Pract* 1996; **46:** 533–535.
Baglin T, Luddington R. Reliability of delayed INR determination: implications for decentralized anticoagulant care with off-site blood sampling. *Br J Haematol* 1997; **96:** 431–434.
Pell JP, McIver B, Stuart P, Malone DN, Alcock J. Comparison of anticoagulant control among patients attending general practice and a hospital anticoagulant clinic. *Br J Gen Pract* 1993; **43:** 152–154.
Fitzmaurice DA, Hobbs FD, Murray ET *et al.* Oral anticoagulation management in primary care with the use of computerized decision support and near-patient testing: a randomized, controlled trial. *Arch Intern Med* 2000; **160:** 2343–2348.
Macgregor SH, Hamley JG, Dunbar JA, Dodd TRP, Cromarty JA. Evaluation of a primary care anticoagulation clinic managed by a pharmacist. *BMJ* 1996; **312:** 560.
British Committee for Standards in Haematology (BCSH). Guidelines on oral anticoagulation: third edition. *Br J Haematol* 1998; **101:** 374–387.
Department of Health. *Investing in General Practice. The New General Medical Services Contract.* London: DH, 2003.
National Collaborating Centre for Chronic Conditions. *Atrial fibrillation: the management of atrial fibrillation. NICE Clinical Guideline 36.* London: NICE, 2006.
Department of Health. *National Service Framework for Coronary Heart Disease.* London: DH, 2000.
www.npsa.nhs.uk
Palareti G, Leali N, Coccheri S *et al.* Bleeding complications of oral anticoagulant treatment: an inception-cohort, prospective collaborative study (ISCOAT). Italian Study on Complications of Oral Anticoagulant Therapy. *Lancet* 1996; **348:** 423–428.
Baglin TP, Keeling DM, Watson HG, British Committee for Standards in Haematology. Guidelines on oral anticoagulation (warfarin): third edition – 2005 update. *Br J Haematol* 2006; **132:** 277–285.

Appendix 7.1. Standard operating procedure for management of POC devices

The POC device must have had approval from the NHS Purchasing and Supply Agency (PASA) as well as *Conformité Européene* (CE) approval. Each device used in the clinic must be named and the serial number recorded. The following issues need to be considered when choosing a device for the clinic and documented within a standard operating procedure (SOP)

Storage arrangements
- Appropriate storage facilities for equipment and reagents (access to constant refrigerated storage space may be required)

Calibration
- Some coagulometers need regular calibration using standardised samples, others have their calibration built into the technology or accomplished by the input of a predetermined code for a new set of reagents. The complexity of the calibration method is a major influence on the degree of staff training
- Potential operator and testing process variables
- POC devices are particularly prone to operator-dependent errors as they may be performed in many different situations with potential for use in uncontrolled circumstances. The more steps involved, the greater the potential for variability in results. Are there many potential operator-dependent variables?
- Each step of the testing process should be documented

Cost
- Cost of quality control material and external assurance scheme
- Cost of technology and reagents
- Cost of training
- Where to order supplies

Maintenance
- Is there a service contract and warranty supplied by the manufacturer?
- If the system fails, is there a back-up system agreed with the local laboratory? (To send venous samples to the lab for INR testing until new system supplied)

Health and safety
- Method of cleaning and disinfection – avoiding cross infection between patients
- Is the equipment for multipatient use with minimal risk of cross infection?

Portability of equipment
- Is the equipment appropriate for home visiting?
- Electrical supply used within the patient's home

Supporting QA schemes
- Internal quality control supplied by the manufacturer
- External quality assurance provided by collaboration with a hospital laboratory should be performed regularly. (In primary care, the practice will need to join a quality assurance scheme to maintain this)
- Liaison with local laboratory for support with training of staff, external quality assurance scheme, to refer patients transferring to the hospital/primary care and if there are any concerns with regard to POC device performance or results

An SOP should record the following:
- Named laboratory personnel
- Equipment ordering and documentation procedures
- Name and serial number of POC device used within the clinic and for home visits
- Name and lot number of reagent strips and internal quality control tests ordered directly from company; name and telephone number of company
- Membership of external quality control scheme
- Log for recording control data and faults, maintenance and repair
- Other equipment used; for example, finger-pricking device, lancets, disposable gloves and sterilising fluid for cleaning machine and mopping up of spilled hazardous waste
- Patient hand-held record books – how INR results are to be recorded with patient ID, and operator ID
- Step-by-step instructions for using the POC device (may be supplied by manufacturer)

Appendix 7.2. Anticoagulation clinic referral form

Patient name: _____

Date of birth: _____/_____/_____

Address: _____

_____

Telephone number: _____

GP referral: Yes ☐   No ☐

If yes, provide name of GP practice: _____

_____

Consultant referral: Yes ☐   No ☐

If yes, name of consultant's hospital: _____

_____

Clinical condition requiring warfarin: _____

_____

Target and range: _____

Concurrent medical conditions: _____

Concurrent medications: _____

Date warfarin commenced: _____/_____/_____

Length of treatment: _____ End date: _____/_____/_____

Current dose: _____

Previous INR results: _____

Signature of clinician: _____ Date: _____

Chapter 8

Medicolegal problems associated with oral anticoagulant services

Professor SJ Machin

Learning outcome

● **The importance of good clinical practice in oral anticoagulation management in terms of professional accountability and potential litigation**

The potential number of medicolegal litigious claims associated with errors in providing oral anticoagulation management is rising. As the therapeutic window of anticoagulant control is relatively narrow, the tendency for the clinical side-effects of under-anticoagulation (recurrent thrombosis) and overdose (spontaneous bleeding) can occur relatively frequently. Such side-effects may arise due to biological variation, patient ignorance or forgetfulness, as well as sub-standard care by the healthcare professionals involved in the delivery of the anticoagulant service. In order to prevent such mistakes, published guidelines are widely available. For example, in the UK, the Haemostasis and Thrombosis Task Force for the British Committee for Standards in Haematology (BCSH) has intermittently (1984, 1990, 1998 and 2005) updated and republished nationally agreed guideline protocols with appropriate levels of evidence. However, despite such protocols, patients are often only within the target international normalised ratio (INR) range 60% of the time and this is still accepted today as a reasonable standard of care.

Negligence

When a patient develops a serious thrombotic or haemorrhagic complication associated with warfarin therapy, the patient – or their carers – sometimes seeks financial compensation through the legal system by trying to prove medical negligence by the healthcare professional involved. This is usually the hospital consultant haematologist responsible for the anticoagulant service, or the GP. As well as having to prove negligence, the plaintiff has also to prove that the negligence involved directly caused the patient harm (causation).

What do we mean by the term negligence? This is generally defined as the medical care provided by the practitioner(s) involved, which fell below the standard level of care that the patient could reasonably expect to have received from a practitioner of similar qalification and training at the date of the alleged incident. For example, if the alleged error was potentially due to the actions of a GP, then these actions would be assessed according to the standard practice of similarly qualified GPs (and not, for example, those of a hospital consultant haematologist/physician specialising in haemostasis and thrombosis). It is an acceptable defence to show that the actions followed would have been similar by a reasonable number (even if a minority) of practitioners of similar qualification, experience and training. This is the Bolam principle which, although recently challenged, is still one of the basic tests of English law, which has to be overcome before negligence can be proved. Obviously, there will be numerous legal nuances that any particular claimant may have to address, but the basic principles of law, that doctors and associated healthcare professionals must remember at all times to account for their actions, are simply expressed above. It is always the responsibility of the plaintiff and his/her legal representatives to prove the alleged particulars of negligence, causation resulting from any negligence and the financial damage, including loss of earnings and projected earnings (known as quantum), that the plaintiff has suffered.

Balance of probabilities

The proof in any civil action, such as a medical negligence claim, is determined by the balance of probabilities test. This requires a greater than 50% chance (51% or more) that the alleged negligent action was responsible for the damage that followed. Therefore, the plaintiff's advisers need to show conclusively, invariably with the aid of written medical expert evidence, preferably supported by contemporary prime review published studies, that the balance of probabilities test is met.

Medical experts used by the plaintiff and defence often disagree over the critical issues, and therefore, in April 1999, the Lord Woolf reforms were introduced to try to speed up the resolution of contentious issues by a series of new recommendations. These allowed for the appointment of a joint expert acceptable to both sides (although this rarely seems to happen) and a pretrial meeting of experts, with a preset agenda, so that matters of agreement and disagreement could be clearly listed. It was hoped that such a definition of issues would lead to earlier settlements of cases and avoidance of costly court trials, with the inevitable delays and anxiety this entails. How successful these reforms have been remains unclear. Obviously, the choice of an appropriate medical expert is critical and,

Table 8.1. Differences between a medical expert and a lawyer

Expert witness	Lawyer
Independent	Partisan
Neutral	Biased
Knows the field	Does not know the field
Witness	Advocate
Gives evidence	Represents a client
Never argues	Argues
Assists the judge	Persuades the judge
Not a hired gun	A hired gun

for the plaintiff, selection of a firm of solicitors who regularly deal with medicolegal claims is essential. However, medical experts must remember to be independent and keep in mind their remit; their role in comparison to that of a lawyer is summarised in Table 8.1, page 63.

Overcoming potential errors within anticoagulation services

Provision of an oral anticoagulation service provides many situations where serious errors may occur. The hospital-based anticoagulant clinic is usually organised by the haematology department, with a consultant haematologist nominally in charge. Good documentation in the clinic, laboratory records of INR testing (now usually computerised) and the patient's own chart and booklet, where clinical INR results and drug dosage changes are listed, are essential to reduce fluctuations in control. A yellow Department of Health patient booklet that has appropriate warnings and records of all clinic attendances, which patients should be issued with and asked to show at all medical consultations, is available free of charge for all clinics. Alternatively, the clinic may issue its own patient record card. Communication with the doctor who initiated treatment, the patient's GP and any other healthcare professional that the patient may consult (for example, a dentist) is also vital. To ensure records are accurate and up to date requires strict local protocols (standard operating procedures in the laboratory), appropriate quality control and regular audit of the overall service provision.

Most cases of medical negligence involving anticoagulation services invariably result from failure or error, often on several occasions, of documentation, communication and/or missing clinic visits. Similar errors may occur in other models of service provision, such as clinics based in general practice (often run by nurse practitioners), pharmacists or patients who self-test (with portable INR machines) and self-dose. The numerous drug interactions that potentiate or inhibit the anticoagulant effects of warfarin provide another source of error. These may not necessarily be prescribed drugs, but also could be a variety of over-the-counter medications (such as St John's wort, which is widely used to combat depression) that are not clearly labelled as causing warfarin interactions. Failure to repeat INR testing about seven days after introducing a drug with known warfarin

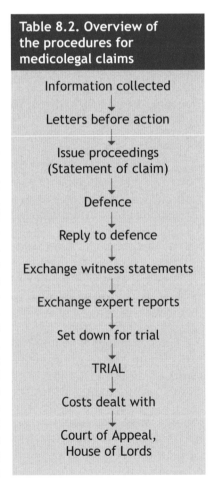

Table 8.2. Overview of the procedures for medicolegal claims

Information collected
↓
Letters before action
↓
Issue proceedings
(Statement of claim)
↓
Defence
↓
Reply to defence
↓
Exchange witness statements
↓
Exchange expert reports
↓
Set down for trial
↓
TRIAL
↓
Costs dealt with
↓
Court of Appeal,
House of Lords

interactions with appropriate dose adjustment puts the patient at potential risk. Again, the fault of such a failure may be complex.

When a patient first starts oral anticoagulant therapy it is important that a responsible member of staff for the clinic counsels the patient carefully about the problems and precautions to be followed. Legally, this is rather similar to a formal signed consent procedure before a planned surgical operation. Ideally, the patient should sign a form indicating that he/she has been appropriately counselled. If such a process has been followed it will be very difficult for the patient to claim at a later date that he/she had not been appropriately warned about potential problems which may arise. When a patient is contemplating legal action, there is a three-year limitation period from the time of the alleged incident (or knowledge of the event, if this occurs at a later time) during which he/she may start legal proceedings. If any action is delayed for more than three years there is a risk that the case may be struck off, due to being time-barred. This rule does not apply to children under the age of 18 years. An overview of procedures that should be followed by a plaintiff contemplating legal action is shown in Table 8.2 (page 64). Some illustrative brief case histories of medical negligence actions that I have experienced (either in my own practice or resulting from being asked to provide a medical opinion) are outlined below.

Case 1

A 76-year-old Caucasian male was admitted as an emergency with an acute upper gastrointestinal bleed. He had been receiving warfarin therapy for five years for atrial fibrillation and carried a yellow national anticoagulant booklet in his pocket. His last INR, five weeks earlier at the hospital clinic, had been 2.7, within his desired therapeutic range of 2.0–3.0. He was maintained on 6 mg of warfarin daily and had been stable on that dose for nine months. On admission his haemoglobin (Hb) was 5.3 g/dl and his INR 9.0 – the rest of his investigations were within normal limits. After resuscitation, including a five-unit blood transfusion and six units of fresh frozen plasma, he required an emergency gastrectomy to control the bleeding. Following stabilisation it transpired that he was receiving no other additional drugs, but the warfarin tablets he had been prescribed four weeks earlier by his pharmacist were 5 mg pink tablets while the typed instructions on the label were to take two 3 mg tablets daily. It transpired that the pharmacist had inadvertently prescribed 5 mg pink tablets instead of 3 mg blue tablets, so that for four weeks the patient had been taking 10 mg instead of 6 mg of warfarin daily. This had caused the prolonged INR and precipitated the acute clinical bleed.

Medicolegal lesson

The basic error in Case 1, above, was obviously with the prescribing pharmacist, whose insurance company admitted full liability. There are four differing strengths of warfarin tablet, which are all specifically colour-coded as 0.5 mg white, 1 mg brown, 3 mg blue and 5 mg pink. Although these coloured tablets are illustrated in the yellow booklet, the patient had followed the instructions on the printed label of the tablet container and had not noticed the change in colour of the prescribed warfarin tablets.

Case 2

A 60-year-old Caucasian male was on long-term warfarin therapy because of a mechanical mitral valve prosthesis, which had been replaced five years earlier. Over this time, his control had been erratic, he had developed hypertension, and had had two episodes of epistaxis and a transient ischaemic attack. As a result of these problems he was being maintained at an INR range of 2.0–3.0 in a district hospital anticoagulant clinic managed by a clinical assistant. He was reviewed every three weeks at the clinic. His previous four clinic visit INRs and warfarin dosages were 2.5, 7 mg; 2.2, 7.5 mg; 2.1, 7.5 mg; and 1.9, 7.5 mg respectively. On his last visit it was noted that he was going on holiday to France for two weeks and would be drinking more alcohol (wine), in modest amounts, than usual. Unfortunately, on the day after his return from holiday (17 days after his last clinic visit) he was admitted as an emergency with an extensive right-middle cerebral-arterial thrombotic stroke. His INR on admission was 1.6.

Medicolegal lesson

After a high court hearing, the defendant hospital trust (on behalf of the clinical assistant and supervising consultant haematologist) was found to be liable of negligence on his last clinic visit before the thrombotic stroke. It was felt that there was a failure to appreciate the risk of a prolonged sub-therapeutic INR in a patient with a metallic valve and, therefore, a high potential incidence of an embolic thrombotic stroke. The constant prescribed dose alone, without increasing the daily maintenance dose of warfarin and/or an earlier clinical visit (even although he was going on holiday), placed the patient in an unacceptable, high-risk situation.

Case 3

A 52-year-old woman was on long-term warfarin therapy for recurrent venous thromboembolism, with a target INR range of 2.0–3.0. Due to a psychiatric disorder of severe agoraphobia she was unable to leave her home and could not attend the hospital clinic. The consultant haematologist had arranged to make domiciliary visits to perform prothrombin time testing and advise of any changes in warfarin dosage by telephone. He usually visited the patient every ten to 12 weeks. At a scheduled visit in March he failed to see her. The patient alleged she telephoned his office on two or three occasions to remind him but got no response. In the meantime, she continued on her maintenance dose of 8 mg daily, as her previous INR three months before had been 2.7. Four months later she contacted her GP because of acute urinary symptoms. He visited her and prescribed an antibiotic for ten days. It is unclear whether the patient mentioned the anticoagulant therapy, or that she had not had an INR test for seven months. One week later, the patient slipped in the garden and knocked her lower back. That evening, because of intense backache, she called out the GP. He visited her, found no abnormalities on examination and prescribed analgesics. Again, there was no written record of her anticoagulant therapy. Twenty-four hours later she developed muscular weakness and paraesthesia in her lower limbs. Following emergency admission to hospital a scan showed an acute spinal haematoma at L1 to L3. Her INR was 9.3. Following warfarin reversal, she had neurosurgical removal of the haematoma but unfortunately was left with severe, permanent neurological damage to her lower limbs.

Medicolegal lesson

The patient began legal proceedings against the consultant haematologist and GP involved in her case. It transpired that the haematologist had been away at the date of planned domiciliary visit and had left no written instructions for his locum. The GP did not specifically consider her long-term warfarin therapy on both visits. In particular, he did not consider the possibility that the acute backache following trauma could be caused by local bleeding associated with her warfarin therapy. In this case the hospital clinic failed to ensure that patients who miss an INR test for more than 12 weeks were contacted and chased up. The GP, on two occasions, did not consider warfarin therapy, possible drug interactions when prescribing an antibiotic, or local progressive internal bleeding as a source of backache. After an exchange of expert reports, the case was settled with the payment split between the two defendants.

Case 4

A 30-year-old West Indian lady was on long-term warfarin therapy, having had a metallic mitral valve fitted three years previously for post-rheumatic mitral stenosis. She was an erratic attendee at the anticoagulant clinic but had been issued with a yellow patient anticoagulant booklet and was maintained on 9 mg warfarin daily with a target INR range of 3.0–4.0. At her previous visit six months earlier, her INR was stable at 3.4. She then attended the clinic again, announcing she was four months pregnant. After considerable discussion and counselling from the haematology and obstetric staff she decided to proceed with an elective termination of pregnancy due to the potential risk of warfarin during the first trimester causing severe fetal malformations, particularly skeletal and neurological defects.

Medicolegal lesson

One year later, solicitors on behalf of the patient issued proceedings against the hospital for failure to specifically warn the patient about the risks of continuing to take warfarin during the first trimester of pregnancy. The haematologist responsible for the service was able to show that the patient had been issued with the yellow booklet and instructed to read it carefully when warfarin therapy was first started. This booklet contains one page dealing with the risks of pregnancy and how patients on warfarin should consult their doctor at the clinic before becoming pregnant. Although clinic staff had not specifically recorded in writing any warnings about pregnancy, the hospital was able to a mount a successful defence because of the implicit warnings in the yellow booklet, which the patient admitted receiving and being told to carefully read it, when treatment was first initiated.

The best approach

As modern medicine becomes more complex, patients have increased expectations about the convenience, promptness and accountability of any treatment they may receive. Long-term oral anticoagulant therapy is no different. Obviously, any patient has the right to know why any particular treatment went wrong, especially if this results in serious illness or permanent disability. The old fashioned attitude of 'the doctor knows best' no longer applies. If a mistake occurs, the best approach is complete frankness and admission of responsibility.

Many hospital trusts have their own risk management group, which will actively internally investigate any reported incident, including meeting the patient and his/her relatives to carefully listen to the specific complaint and answer points of contention. If any error is found, admission of fault is the best policy and the trust's legal representatives should be instructed to negotiate a suitable financial settlement. Unfortunately, some patients have difficulty in accepting that certain complications are unavoidable and are a known risk of the treatment plan. In such cases the doctor's actions must be fully supported.

Lengthy, expensive legal actions should be avoided if at all possible and further potential errors should be prevented by the improvement of local protocols, using clinical governance and internal audit. Any healthcare professional involved in the delivery or organisation of an oral anticoagulant service must be aware of the potential medicolegal problems that may develop and, hopefully, by being vigilant, prevent expensive lawsuits and also improve the standard of their clinical practice.

Summary

- As the therapeutic window of anticoagulant control is relatively narrow, clinical side-effects can occur relatively frequently. Therefore, the potential number of medico-legal litigious claims associated with errors in providing oral anticoagulation management is rising.
- Clinical outcomes can be due to patient ignorance, forgetfulness or sub-standard care by the health professionals involved in the delivery of the anticoagulant service.
- Patients or their carers often seek financial compensation through the legal system by trying to prove medical negligence by the healthcare professional involved.
- If an alleged error was potentially due to the actions of a GP, then these actions would be assessed according to the standard practice of a similarly qualified GP and

not, for example, those of a hospital consultant haematologist/physician specialising in haemostasis and thrombosis (Bolam principle).

● Methods of overcoming potential litigation include:

1. Good documentation in the clinic, laboratory records of international normalisd ratio (INR) testing and the patient's own booklet where clinical INR results and drug dosage changes are listed

2. Communication between the doctor who initiated treatment, the patient's GP and any other healthcare professional the patient may consult (for example, a dentist)

3. Strict local protocols, appropriate quality control and regular audit of the overall service provision.

● For patients who self-dose it is important that there is an agreed algorithm for dose changes, retesting intervals and when to urgently attend or contact the main clinic.

● It is important that the responsible professional counsels the patient carefully about the problems and precautions that should be followed when first starting oral anti-coagulant therapy. Legally, this is similar to a formal signed consent procedure before a planned surgical operation.

● Any healthcare professional involved in the management of oral anticoagulation must be aware of the potential medicolegal problems and that frank admission of any fault is the best policy. The trust's legal representatives should be instructed to negotiate a suitable financial settlement.

Further reading
British Committee for Standards in Haematology (BCSH). Guidelines on oral anticoagulation: third edition. *Br J Haematol* 1998; **101:** 374–387.
Band C, Solan M, Harper P. *The expert in court – a practical guide*. Guildford: Shaw & Sons Ltd, 1997.

Chapter 9

The economics of antithrombotic therapy for stroke prevention and anticoagulation clinics

Dr S Jowett

Professor J Raftery

Learning outcomes

- **Cost-effectiveness issues from both societal and NHS perspectives**
- **Funding issues related to oral anticoagulation management**
- **Sources of funding for primary care anticoagulation clinics**
- **Issues to be addressed when applying for funding**

This chapter reviews two main issues and is separated into two distinct parts.

Part 1: The case for antithrombotic therapy for patients with non-rheumatic atrial fibrillation and issues around patient perspectives and patient self-monitoring are discussed.
Part 2: Detailed costing required at practice level is investigated and funding issues, including sources of funding, examined.

Part 1. The economics of antithrombotic therapy for stroke prevention

Introduction

The economics of antithrombotic therapy provide a good example of many of the difficult issues raised in economic evaluations associated with healthcare, as follows:

- How much reliance to place on clinical trial estimates of the effectiveness of different treatments
- Which perspective to take in both costing and in measuring and valuing benefits
- Which benefits (clinical, patient-oriented, risks) to include, over what time period
- What likely cost 'offsets', including savings due to events, could be averted within different scales of operation (big hospital clinics, primary care or self-monitoring)
- How we should assess new technologies and new policies, both of which are rapidly evolving.

Epidemiology of stroke prevention

Early exploration of the risk factors for stroke came from the long-running Framingham Heart Study in the USA, which first identified atrial fibrillation (AF) as a risk factor for stroke (and coined the term 'risk factor'). Four main independent risk factors were initially identified for stroke: hypertension, coronary heart disease (CHD), heart failure, and AF. Some 30 other risk factors have been added since. The relative importance of these risk factors can be assessed in different ways. In terms of relative risk of stroke, AF has a value of 5, exceeded only by having had a previous stroke (relative risk 9–15) or a transient ischaemic attack (7). Population attributable risk fraction shows the percentage of strokes attributable to each risk factor (Table 9.1), indicating that AF is particularly important among the higher age groups, especially those aged 80–89 years.

Number of strokes to be expected in a typical practice

We can make some estimates of the expected numbers of AF patients as follows. With a 3–6% prevalence of AF in patients aged 65 and over, who comprise 20% of the population, then we have between 72 and 144 AF patients in a practice of 12,000 patients. If 33–50% are suitable for antithrombotic therapy, then this is equivalent to 24–72 patients.

Approximately 20% of all strokes occur among patients with AF. On the basis of a predicted two strokes per 1,000 population per annum, in a general practice with 12,000 people, we could expect around 24 strokes each year, with around five of these in AF patients.

Preferred treatment

The choice of treatment between oral anticoagulation and antiplatelet therapy is controversial. A meta-analysis by Hart *et al* in 1999 favoured warfarin over aspirin and placebo, while a more recent systematic review by Taylor *et al* concluded that there was considerable uncertainty about the value of long-term anticoagulation compared with

Table 9.1. Population attributable risk fractions for four risk factors for stroke (%)

Age group	60-69	70-79	80-89
Hypertension	53	49	33
CHD	12	13	0
Cardiac failure	12	18	19
Atrial fibrillation	3	10	24

Source: Wade DT. Stroke (acute cerebrovascular disease). In: Stevens A, Raftery J (eds). *Health care needs assessment*. Oxford: Radcliffe Medical Press, 1993: 178.

antiplatelet treatment. It suggested that the main trial favouring anticoagulation was methodologically weak. The results of the BAFTA trial conducted by Mant *et al* in 2007 investigated the optimal treatment in AF patients aged 75, as this subgroup had been previously under-represented in treatment trials. The results supported the use of anti-coagulation in this patient group, unless there were contraindications or patients felt the inconvenience outweighed the benefits. The most recent clinical guidelines, pro-duced by the National Institute for Health and Clinical Excellence (NICE) in 2006, rec-ommended that stroke risk be used to inform the final decision, and for moderate risk patients, they acknowledge the lack of clear-cut evidence, and advocate decision-making at an individual patient level.

Numbers needed to treat for oral anticoagulation

The one year numbers needed to treat (NNTs) for anticoagulation and stroke have been estimated to be 37 for primary prevention and 12 for secondary prevention for adjusted-dose warfarin compared with placebo.

Measurable outcomes

No agreement exists on the relevant outcome to be measured (see Chapter 6). Candidates include: the percentage of patients in the international normalised ratio (INR) range; the time spent in the INR range; strokes prevented; deaths prevented; life-years gained; and quality-adjusted life-years (QALYs).

Time in therapeutic range

Each measure has merits depending on perspective. For clinicians using anticoagula-tion therapy, the percentage of patients in the INR range may be a good indicator for comparing two services, such as community versus hospital clinics.

A focus on INR control as proxy or intermediate outcome would enable us to take a similar approach as in the evaluation of screening programmes (that is, cost per case detected). However, we do not know how important it is to maintain patients with INR by time.

Stroke and adverse events

Most studies have focused on the number of strokes prevented as the primary outcome. This could be seen as a more public or social outcome (Table 9.2, page 73). Both the meta-analysis by Hart *et al* in 1999 and the systematic review by Taylor *et al* in 2001 considered strokes prevented.

They found significantly more adverse events (intracranial bleeds) in those treated with warfarin; however, these results were not borne out in the BAFTA trial, where there was no significant difference in event rates between the warfarin and aspirin arms of the study. The effects of adverse events on patients' quality of life have only received limited exploration.

Strokes	No therapy	Aspirin	Warfarin	Gain: No therapy - aspirin	Gain: Warfarin - aspirin
Low risk	10	8	4	2	4
Medium risk	35	28	14	7	14
High risk	60	48	24	12	24
Secondary prevention	120	96	48	24	48

Table 9.2. Effects of anticoagulation on 1,000 patients at different levels of risk in terms of strokes prevented

Source: Antithrombotics and stroke in AF. *Bandolier*, December 1999, 70-72. www.jr2.ox.ac.uk/Bandolier

Deaths averted

Hart *et al's* meta-analysis showed a significant decline in all-cause mortality for warfarin relative to placebo. No differences in mortality could be discerned between warfarin and aspirin, partly due to the lack of power in the clinical trials to detect any such differences.

Life-years gained and QALYs

From a public health or societal perspective, the more appropriate goal may be life-years or QALYs. Given that stroke and AF are diseases of the elderly, the question of how many years might be generated from oral anticoagulation treatment is important. If those years might not be of high quality of life, then QALYs are required. Such generic outcome measures would enable different programmes to be compared; no trial of antithrombotic therapy has used such measures.

The life-years generated from stroke prevention in the elderly are likely to be relatively few in general, due to the limited life expectancy of this age group. Ideally for economic analysis one would want, in addition to any gain in life-years, the value the population would place on the health states in which those additional life-years were lived. These could be used to provide the cost per QALY from a societal perspective. There is considerable disagreement in the literature as to how to measure the health states and whether the values should be those of the ill or the well. One study by Robinson *et al* in 2001 of utilities in stroke, major bleed and anticoagulation based on a relatively small sample (57) of AF patients in the UK (Table 9.3, page 74) demonstrated a number of interesting findings:

● Health state values varied as expected with the severity of stroke
● There was a lot of individual variation, with many ranking major stroke as equal to death
● A major bleed (gastrointestinal bleed) results in lower quality of life for a short period of time

Table 9.3. Mean (median) health state valuations from sample of AF patients (1.0 = perfect health)				
Mild stroke	Severe stroke	Major bleed	Warfarin (GP)	Warfarin (hospital)
0.64 (0.68)	0.19 (0)	0.84 (0.88)	0.95 (0.99)	0.94 (0.98)

Source: Robinson A, Thomson R, Parkin D, Sudlow M, Eccles M. How patients with atrial fibrillation value different health outcomes: a standard gamble study. *J Health Serv Res Policy* 2001: **6**: 92-98.

● Health states related to being on warfarin and attending a hospital or GP clinic were close to 1.0, suggesting that the therapy does not significantly lower people's quality of life.

It should be noted that this was a sample of ill people, so that a sample of well people might have yielded different values. For publicly funded services, according to economic theory, it is the values of the well rather than the ill that should determine decisions, and this is the approach taken by NICE. Patient perceptions of risk are critical to decisions to accept anticoagulation therapy. How patients value risk is an issue which has received almost no attention in the debate around anticoagulation therapy. Patients on anticoagulation therapy are implicitly or explicitly trading off reduced risks from future stroke against increased ongoing risks of adverse events. The degree to which patients understand these trade-offs is a critical issue to be researched and used in assessing cost-effectiveness. The overall conclusion on outcomes is that the literature has focused almost entirely on strokes averted and to a lesser extent on mortality, with no data available on life-years or QALYs generated. Risk and adverse events have been neglected in assessing benefits.

Costs

Healthcare economics are concerned with a wide definition of costs, including those falling on the NHS, patients, and society. Most guidelines for economic evaluation follow welfare economics and argue for a societal perspective in which all costs are taken into account. In practice, however, most UK studies take the perspective of the payer, usually the NHS or the public sector. The costs of stroke, however, extend well beyond the health service and should include costs to local authorities in relation to both personal social services and residential and nursing care. Costs may be borne by patients and their families due to charges for some social services but mainly in relation to caring by relatives. Estimates of the costs to the NHS of anticoagulation management and the costs of strokes averted are discussed below. Very few data are available on the costs to patients and carers.

Unit costs of anticoagulation have put consultant-led hospital anticoagulation management at around £100. In terms of primary care costs, Parry *et al* showed that oral anticoagulation management was at least as effective as hospital care but the cost per patient is higher than hospital outpatient care (£160 per patient per annum against

£88) on average (1996/97 prices). However, the cost per patient was less in bigger practices and fell to roughly the level of hospital care when the number of patients requiring treatment was around 40. The cost of patient self-management of warfarin will be discussed in detail later in the chapter. Aspirin costs can be taken as being close to zero, but some costs may be entailed in ensuring compliance and monitoring results.

Cost of strokes prevented

Arguably, what matters is not gross but net cost. Net cost would include the savings due to strokes averted. The main NHS cost of strokes is related to hospital admissions. The costs per emergency stroke by type of stroke, as defined by the healthcare resource group (HRG) are summarised in Table 9.4. For the non-transient stroke group A22Z, the mean cost is £2,261. However, these data exclude the small number of very long stay patients, some of whom spend months in hospital. Additional costs would be imposed, particularly for those disabled post-stroke, some of whom would require nursing home care, which costs from £300 to £500 per week.

Could oral anticoagulation therapy be cost-neutral?

Using the NNTs of 37 and 12 for all and high risk, and taking the cost of anticoagulation at £100 per patient per annum, then the cost would be £3,700 per stroke for primary prevention and £1,200 for secondary prevention, each year. If the cost per patient anticoagulated was doubled due to primary care clinics or self-management, the total costs of the programme would double.

As shown above, the hospital cost of each stroke patient admitted is around £2,000. The additional costs of rehabilitation, and family or nursing home care might roughly double this. Overall, the cost of an oral anticoagulation therapy programme would be roughly offset if one stroke was prevented each year, which seems likely. However, an individual practice might not save money as reductions in the numbers admitted to hospitals or nursing homes will not translate into savings, at least in the short term.

Table 9.4. Number and cost of emergency stroke admissions to NHS acute hospitals 2006–2007

HRG		No. FCEs	Mean £	Average length of stay (days)
A29Z	Transient ischaemic attack	17,421	756	3
A22Z	Non-transient stroke or cerebrovascular accident, nervous system infections or encephalopathy	104,171	2,261	10

Source: NHS Reference costs, 2006/07. HRG = healthcare resource group. FCE = finished consultant episode

Table 9.5. Cost per stroke prevented by intervention	
Intervention	**Cost per stroke prevented (£)**
Blood pressure: tight control of hypertension	£18,095-110,476
Anticoagulation of eligible AF patients	£3,800
Aspirin for patients with CHD or AF not on warfarin	£164
Aspirin post-stroke	£62
Carotid endarterectomy	£27,700

Source: Mant J, Wade D. Stroke. In: Stevens A, Raftery J, Mant J (eds). *Health care needs assessment: updated*. Oxford: Radcliffe Medical Press, 2002. AF = atrial fibrillation. CHD = coronary heart disease

The cost-effectiveness of stroke prevention

The best available attempt at estimating the cost-effectiveness of measures to prevent stroke is shown in Table 9.5, which shows that anticoagulation of eligible AF patients is £3,800 per stroke prevented. This is more than for the use of aspirin, either for coronary heart disease treatment or treatment of AF, but is considerably less than for blood pressure control or carotid endarterectomy.

Patient self-management

The economic evaluation conducted by Jowett *et al* alongside the SMART study trial demonstrated the anticoagulation-related costs over 12 months associated with patient self-management (PSM) (£382) were greater than those for routine hospital or GP care (£90). The cost of a point-of-care (POC) device is currently £400 (plus VAT), which is approximately £160 per year if it lasts three years (£100 a year over five years). The primary additional cost is the test strips at £2.50 per test, and testing was every two weeks, more often if dosage changes were required. The study also took into account training, patient assessment visits, internal quality control and consumables. Additional NHS costs for primary and secondary care visits for minor and serious adverse events did not differ greatly between the two arms. As QALYs were very similar in the two trial arms, the results suggested that PSM would not be a cost-effective use of NHS resources.

Uncertainties

Matters of debate include:
● The relative merits of aspirin and warfarin
● The valuation of adverse events and risk by patients
● The future role of the hospital (such as outreach, IT communication, patient-centred approaches)

- The future role of primary care trusts (PCTs) – shared oral anticoagulation therapy clinics
- Changes in technology for anticoagulation management – cheaper POC testing; enabling patients to adjust dosage; internet feedback on INR adjustments; cheaper self-monitoring kits, new less risky anticoagulants (such as dabigatran).

Conclusions

Antithrombotic therapy offers scope for sizeable reductions in stroke risk but only as one part of stroke strategy. The best strategies depend on the number of AF patients suitable for therapy in a practice or PCT, their ages, and the convenience of practices to patients compared to hospital services.

While aspirin is in general likely to be the least costly, its merits relative to warfarin remain contentious. For anticoagulation therapy, hospital is likely to be the cheapest, but may be less clinically effective and more inconvenient for patients. Primary care is likely to be at least as good clinically but more expensive than hospital therapy, unless the primary care anticoagulation clinic has more than 40 patients. For the purposes of organising a clinic, what matters is the total number of patients requiring anticoagulation, regardless of whether this is due to AF, deep vein thrombosis or pulmonary embolism. Estimation of cost-effectiveness is curtailed by lack of outcomes data in terms of life-years or QALYs. Cost data tend to be confined to the NHS. Patient self-monitoring may become more common, but at a higher cost, which may be met wholly or in part by patients' contributions.

For any kind of oral anticoagulation management, it will be important to collect an agreed minimum data set for monitoring (Chapter 6). It will also be necessary in primary care strategies to have quality assurance of INR measuring equipment.

Finally, the importance of including patients' values regarding disadvantages/benefits needs to be emphasised. The values placed by patients on convenience, risk and adverse events may be critical to the economic evaluation of antithrombotic therapy.

Summary

- Approximately 20% of all strokes occur among patients with atrial fibrillation (AF) and around 80% of these may be prevented by antithrombotic therapy.
- In a general practice with 12,000 people, we could expect around 24 strokes each year, with around five of these in AF patients.
- The one year numbers needed to treat (NNTs) for anticoagulation and stroke are 37 for primary prevention and 12 for secondary prevention for adjusted-dose warfarin compared with placebo.
- No agreement exists on the relevant outcome to be measured (Chapter 6).
- Most studies have focused on the number of strokes prevented, which is a more public or social outcome, but from a public health or societal perspective the more appropriate goal may be life-years or quality-adjusted life-years (QALYs).
- For economic analysis one would want, in addition to any gain in life-years, the value the population would place on the health states in which those additional life-years were lived.

- The costs of strokes extend well beyond the health service and should include costs to local authorities in relation to both personal social services and residential and nursing care.
- For the most common stroke group A22Z, the mean cost is £2,261. However, these data exclude the small number of very long stay patients, some of whom spend months in hospital.
- Overall, the cost of an oral anticoagulation therapy programme would be roughly offset if one stroke was prevented each year. However, an individual practice might not save money as reductions in the numbers admitted to hospitals or nursing homes will not translate into savings, at least in the short term.
- Primary care is likely to be clinically at least as good but more expensive than hospital care, unless the primary care anticoagulation clinic has more than 40 patients. Therefore, for the purposes of organising a clinic, what matters is the total number of patients requiring anticoagulation, regardless of whether this is due to AF, deep vein thrombosis or pulmonary embolism.

Part 2. Funding issues
Introduction
Primary care teams are now increasingly becoming aware of the importance of anticoagulation services, for reasons that have been previously outlined. As part of the General Medical Services (GMS) contract, the Quality and Outcomes Framework (QOF), an annual reward and incentive programme for primary care, encourages the identification of patients with AF, the keeping of an AF register, and treatment with anticoagulant or antiplatelet therapy. An increasing number of patients with AF are receiving anticoagulation therapy and the proportion of AF patients out of the total number of patients who are anticoagulated (for example, patients with mechanical heart valves, pulmonary embolus or deep vein thrombosis) has also increased.

The need to ensure that these patients are adequately monitored and controlled places a burden on the current anticoagulation monitoring services. PCTs are also aware of the associated increased costs, and requests received from NHS trusts for additional funding.

There may be concerns about the risks to patients of haemorrhage when the degree of control is not satisfactory and this may lead to reluctance within primary care to initiate anticoagulation therapy. Older people may be at a particular risk because monitoring and control may be difficult in this age group. The costs to patients of anticoagulation in terms of time, travel, and inconvenience must not be ignored. As we have seen, the quality of control is essential – otherwise anticoagulation therapy may be more harmful than beneficial.

Practices are, therefore, faced with a dilemma and a set of difficult issues to resolve. The practice will need to work through the following set of questions.

- Does the practice have an overall strategy for the prevention and treatment of stroke?
- Does anticoagulation of patients who have AF provide a worthwhile reduction in the risk of stroke? As we have seen, there is a two-thirds reduction of risk (three strokes prevented per year in a practice of size 12,000 at a neutral cost).

- How are oral anticoagulation management services best provided? Hospital antico-agulation monitoring services are already under strain and studies have shown that the quality of control is less than ideal. Hospital-based services may be more cost-efficient, but high-quality control of INR is essential. Quality of control is influenced by the ease with which patients can access the service; long waits at a hospital-based clinic that is difficult to access will be not be helpful to patients, particularly older patients.
- Is the practice willing and able to develop practice-based anticoagulation services?

Once the practice has answered these questions and established that there is a need to develop an oral anticoagulation service, a decision on how this can be taken forward must then be made.

How to approach the development of oral anticoagulation services

The primary care team will need to decide what approach it will take to developing the anticoagulation service and how it will obtain the necessary funds. It is suggested that the development of anticoagulation services should be within the context of the PCT Health Improvement Programme. Although this approach cannot guarantee that additional funding will be forthcoming, it does enable the PCT to identify how the allocation of additional resources to the practice will contribute to the achievement of its health improvement targets. Decentralisation of service provision has been encouraged through the enhanced services payment system within the new GMS contract for primary care. There is a nationally agreed service specification, and depending on the level of service provided, primary care service providers can generate revenue by managing patients receiving anticoagulation. National Enhanced Services were introduced in April 2004 as part of the new GMS contract.

Identify and quantify the benefits

One possible approach is the identification and quantification of the benefits of establishing the anticoagulation service in terms of reduction in the number of deaths and disability from strokes, and improvement in quality of life. For example, a practice with 12,000 patients would expect 24 strokes per year, and five of these in patients with atrial fibrillation; three strokes per year could be averted.

Determine the numbers of patients who are likely to require anticoagulation

As stated earlier in the chapter, prevalence estimates could be used to determine the numbers of patients who may need anticoagulation. For example, the prevalence of AF is 3–6% in people aged over 65 years and 30–50% of these may be suitable for anticoagulation; therefore, in a practice with 12,000 patients there would be between 24 and 72 people suitable for anticoagulation management.

Identify the possible options for how anticoagulation services can be provided

There are a number of possibilities:
- Totally hospital-based
- Practice-based, such as POC testing within the practice
- Hybrid; for example, phlebotomy and dosing at the practice – INR test and interpretation at the hospital
- Patient self-monitoring/management.

The number of patients who are likely to be treated may influence the choice. NHS costs can be minimised if the patient numbers are in excess of 40 (this number will include patients anticoagulated for indications other than chronic AF). For practices where the number of patients is likely to be small, a hospital-based or 'hybrid' model may be appropriate. For larger practices, a model that is totally practice-based might be feasible. However, there may be scope for smaller practices to collaborate and to share the provision of anticoagulation management services; this approach could be facilitated by the PCT (a 'hub and spoke' model). The disadvantage of this approach is that some of the benefits of the provision of local, accessible services based within the community may be lost. The service model that the practice chooses will need to correspond to one of the four service levels included within the new GMS contract, because this is how the practice will be funded by the PCT. These are shown in Table 9.6. The practice will need to decide which model most meets local health needs and is the most cost-effective, taking into account local circumstances and the costs to the practice of providing the service.

Calculate the costs of each option

An approximate annual cost of organising anticoagulation management totally within the practice can be estimated. Information is required on the proposed clinic set-up, and all the component parts required for the clinic, each of which will have a unit cost. First, information is required on how the clinic is to be organised and the number of patients expected:

Table 9.6 GMS contract service levels (2003-04 prices)

Level	Model	Amount (£)
1	Laboratory outreach sampling, test and dose	6-10
2	HA, trust or other externally funded phlebotomist, pharmacist etc, practice sample, laboratory test, practice dosing	75-100
3	Practice-funded phlebotomist, pharmacist etc, practice sample, laboratory test, practice dosing	80-110
4	Practice-funded phlebotomist or pharmacist etc, practice sample, practice test, practice dosing	85-120

Prices uprated by 3.225% in 2004-05 and again in 2005-06. GMS = General Medical Services

- Number of patients on anticoagulation and attending the clinic
- Estimates of the number of new patients and patients discontinuing treatment (or dying) over a 12-month period
- Average number of visits per patient in 12 months.

This information will establish the overall number of clinic visits expected in a 12-month period. Further information on clinic organisation is then required:

- Number of clinics per week
- Estimated length of each clinic
- Time per appointment for established patients
- Time per appointment for new patients (in order to deliver patient education)
- Expected additional input from medical (for example, GP) and clerical staff.

The chief costs to be taken into account when running a clinic are as follows:

- Consumables – blood testing strips, lancets, and gloves
- Equipment – POC device, computer, software
- Premises – heating, lighting, rent and so on (overheads)
- Internal quality control and membership of the UK National External Quality Assessment Service
- Other costs, such as training.

These costs can be categorised as variable, fixed and semi-fixed costs. Variable costs are those incurred at every patient attendance, namely consumable costs. The key cost here is that of the test strips. Semi-fixed costs increase with the number of clinics required by a practice and include staff costs, staff training, overheads and internal quality control. As the number of clinics required a week increases, then additional costs are incurred. For example, an additional practice nurse may be required to run the clinic, adding to both staff costs and training costs. Additional clinics will incur greater premises costs; for example, heating, lighting and rent of the room. Fixed costs are those that are incurred irrespective of the volume of patients through the clinic, namely equipment costs. The cost is amortised over the life of the equipment at a discount rate of 3.5% per annum, giving an equivalent annual cost. An additional fixed cost is external quality control, which is a set annual amount. Finally, a further cost to be considered if that of domiciliary visits. If these visits are undertaken by a member of practice staff (such as a practice nurse) then additional costs are incurred in the form of additional time required (additional staff costs) and travel expenses.

Once all this information is available, it can be entered into a costing model, which is designed to calculate total cost per patient per year and cost per patient visit (see www.anticoagulation.org.uk). The range of costs per patient per year can vary widely depending on the number of patients within the programme and how the clinic is configured, but are roughly in the region of £100 to £150 a year, although can be greater if the patient numbers are low. The costs of a service that is totally hospital-based have been estimated to be £100 per patient per year. However, this will vary locally, and will depend on the actual prices that a particular trust charges.

Compare the costs and benefits of each option

It is important that a decision is made on what is most appropriate for the local circumstances. One factor that may be important in influencing the model that is chosen is the number of patients per year that are to be managed.

Sources of funds for the development of anticoagulation services

PCTs are responsible for commissioning health services and the allocation of NHS resources to meet local health needs. The practice will, therefore, need to work closely with its PCT in order to gain access to the funding that will be required to establish anticoagulation services.

The new GMS contract – National Enhanced Services

Anticoagulation management services are included in the list of National Enhanced Services within the new GMS contract and this is the mechanism for funding these services in primary care (along with the Personal Medical Services contract). PCTs are able to commission enhanced services from practices if they believe that these will meet local needs. The purpose of enhanced services is to:
● Improve patient care for all patients and for specific vulnerable groups
● Improve patient choice
● Aid the shift of services (and resources) from secondary to primary care.

The PCT is required to take account of these aims when commissioning anticoagulation services and considering whether to invest in general practice.

This funding mechanism replaces others that might have been used in the past, such as local development schemes, improving primary care incentive schemes and the national framework for the provision of secondary care within general practice. PCTs are required to spend minimum levels of money on enhanced services in primary care; however, they are able to invest greater levels of funding if required to meet local needs. There are no new sources of funding for this and any additional money must come from the PCT's unified budget.

Summary

● Practices are faced with a dilemma and a set of difficult issues to resolve. The practice will need to work through the following set of questions:
    – Does the practice have an overall strategy for the prevention and treatment of stroke?
    – Does anticoagulation of patients who have atrial fibrillation (AF) provide a worthwhile reduction in the risk of stroke?
    – How are oral anticoagulation management services best provided? Is the practice willing and able to develop practice-based anticoagulation services?
● Within the context of the primary care trust (PCT) local delivery plan, the PCT will need to identify how the allocation of additional resources to the practice will contribute to the achievement of its health improvement targets by:

- Identifying and quantifying the benefits of establishing the anticoagulation service in terms of reduction in the number of deaths and disability from strokes, and improvement in quality of life
- Determining the numbers of patients likely to require anticoagulation using prevalence estimates
- Identifying the possible options for how anticoagulation services can be provided
- Calculating the costs of each option
- Comparing the costs and benefits of each option, and deciding on what is most appropriate for the local circumstances.

● The practice will need to develop and write a proposal or action plan to include the development of a clinical protocol that describes how the service will operate, how patients will be managed and what clinical audit will be undertaken.

● The practice will need to work closely with its PCT in order to gain access to the funding that will be required to establish anticoagulation services.

● The main funding source is through the enhanced services payment system within the new GMS contract for primary care.

Further reading

Ebrahim S, Hardwood R. *Stroke: Epidemiology, evidence and clinical practice*, 2nd edn. Oxford: Oxford University Press, 1999.

Sudlow M, Thomson R, Thwaites B, Rodsers H, Kenny RA. Prevalence of atrial fibrillation and eligibility for anticoagulants in the community. *Lancet* 1998; **352**: 1167–1171.

Wade DT. Stroke (acute cerebrovascular disease). In: Stevens A, Raftery J (eds). *Health care needs assessment*. Oxford: Radcliffe Medical Press, 1993.

Antithrombotics and stroke in AF. Bandolier, 1999, 70–72. www.jr2.ox.ac.uk/Bandolier

Gage RF, Cardinalli AB, Albers GW, Owen DK. Cost effectiveness of warfarin with aspirin for prophylaxis of stroke in patients with non valvular atrial fibrillation. *JAMA* 1995; **274**: 1839–1845.

Taylor FC, Gray A, Cohen H *et al.* Costs and effectiveness of a nurse specialist anticoagulant service. *J Clin Pathology* 1997; **50**: 823–828.

Taylor F, Cohen H, Ebrahim S. Systematic review of long term anticoagulation or antiplatelet treatment in patients with non rheumatic atrial fibrillation. *BMJ* 2001; **322**: 321–326.

Robinson A, Thomson R, Parkin D, Sudlow M, Eccles M. How patients with atrial fibrillation value different health outcomes: a standard gamble study. *J Health Serv Res Policy* 2001; **6**: 92–98.

Parry D, Fitzmaurice, D, Raftery J. Anticoagulation management in primary care: a trial based economic evaluation. *Brit J Haematol* 2000; **111**: 530–533.

Wolf PA, D'Agostino RB, Belanger AJ, Kannel WB. Probability of a stroke: a risk profile from the Framingham study. *Stroke* 1991; **22**: 312–318.

Hart RG, Benavente O, McBride R, Pearce LA. Antithrombotic therapy to prevent stroke in patients with atrial fibrillation: a meta analysis. *Ann Int Med* 1999; **131**: 429–501.

NHS Reference costs, 2006/07. London: Department of Health, 2008.

Mant J, Wade D. Stroke. In: Stevens A, Raftery J, Mant J (eds). *Health care needs assessment: updated*. Oxford: Radcliffe Medical Press, 2002.

Mant J, Hobbs FDR, Fletcher K *et al.* Warfarin versus aspirin for stroke prevention in an elderly population with atrial fibrillation (the Birmingham Atrial Fibrillation treatment of the Aged Study, BAFTA): a randomised controlled trial. *Lancet* 2007; **370**: 493–503.

National Collaborating Centre for Chronic Conditions. Atrial fibrillation: national clinical guideline for management in primary and secondary care. London: Royal College of Physicians, 2006.

Jowett SM, Bryan S, Murray E *et al.* Patient self-management of anticoagulation therapy: a trial-based cost-effectiveness analysis. *Br J Haematol* 2006; **134**: 632–639.

Lip GYH, Beevers DG, Coope JR. ABC of Atrial Fibrillation: Atrial fibrillation in general and hospital practice. *BMJ* 1996; **312**: 175–178.

Lip GYH, Lowe GDO. ABC of Atrial Fibrillation: Antithrombotic treatment for Atrial fibrillation. *BMJ* 1996; **312**: 45-49.

Pell JP, McIver B, Malone DNS, Alcock J. Comparison of anti-coagulation control among patients attending general practice and a hospital anti-coagulation clinic. *Br J Gen Pract* 1993; **43**: 152–154.

Kannel WB, Abbott RD, Savage DD, McNamara PM. Epidemiological features of the Framingham study. *N Engl J Med* 1982; **306**: 1018–1022.

Department of Health. Investing in General Practice. The New General Medical Services Contract. London: Department of Health, 2003.

British Medical Association. National enhanced service – anti-coagulation monitoring. http://www.bma.org.uk/

Chapter 10

Patient self-management of oral anticoagulation

Dr ET Murray

Professor DA Fitzmaurice

Learning outcomes

- **Background to patient self-management for oral anticoagulation**
- **Trial data to support patient self-management**

In recent years, with the development of point-of-care testing (POCT) for international normalised ratio (INR) testing, there has been a move towards patients measuring their own INRs and adjusting their own dosage of anticoagulant. Problems that are inherent to clinic models have provided the impetus for the move towards patient self-management (PSM), as patients have demanded more autonomy and control over their condition. There are potentially two levels at which patients' can manage their anticoagulation therapy: self-testing and self-management.

Patient self-testing

The patient is responsible for testing their INR at home using capillary sampling and a point-of-care (POC) testing device, though dosing of warfarin and frequency of testing are advised by the healthcare professional clinically responsible for their management. Internal quality control (IQC), external quality assessment (EQA), and general maintenance of the POC device and test strips can be the responsibility of either the patient or healthcare professional, but this has to be agreed before patient self-testing (PST) commences.

Patient self-management

The patient is responsible for testing their INR at home using capillary sampling and a POC device and also for dosing of warfarin and frequency of testing, with support from the healthcare professional clinically responsible, according to an agreed contract. The patient is seen at agreed intervals to assess their INR control and offer advice.

IQC and EQA and general maintenance of the POC device and test strips can again be the responsibility of either the patient or the healthcare professional, agreed before PSM commences. This may be included in the follow-up consultation.

Patient self-testing/management of oral anticoagulation can be seen as a progression from the primary care POC anticoagulation model and is comparable to home glucose monitoring using a portable glucometer.

While convenience and patient autonomy are undoubtedly important, the relative clinical safety and effectiveness of PSM in comparison to existing models of care must be established before recommendations can be made regarding its wider implementation.

The evidence

The most recent meta-analysis and systematic review, which superseded two previous reviews, included 14 randomised, controlled trials (RCTs) of self-monitoring, with a total of 3,049 participants.[1]

It comprised both adult and paediatric studies and information was collected on primary outcome measures, INR control and bleeding or thrombotic events, secondary outcomes of frequency of testing, minor bleeds and dropout rate. In addition to this, disease characteristics, training undertaken, self-dosing methods and number of participants refusing to self-manage were also investigated. Nine of the trials, three from the UK, had been published within the previous three years of the review and consequently had not been included in previous reviews. There were no studies from the earlier reviews not included in the most recent review.

Self-testing and self-management was found to be associated with a significant one-third reduction in major haemorrhage, and a non-significant reduction in the self-management group alone. A significant reduction in death was noted in the self-management group of studies (p=0.03). The interpretation of the review was positive in terms of the quality of oral anticoagulation management through self-management but suggested that self-monitoring is not feasible for all patients, in that patients need to be identified carefully and trained.

The authors did state limitations to the review, in that variability of care in control groups potentially affected the comparisons. It could be argued, therefore, that the positive conclusions deduced with regard to self-monitoring rely on the imbalance of studies from outside the UK, where worse INR control is seen for routine care. It may, therefore, not be appropriate to apply the same conclusions to the UK.

This opinion was reinforced in another systematic review, updated for the UK guidelines for self-management of oral anticoagulation.[2] This review included cohort and observational studies as well as RCTs up to 2003 and found poor therapeutic control within other healthcare systems where physician office or GP testing was routine practice and anticoagulation hospital clinics were not as well established or widespread as they are in the UK. Consequently, improvement in therapeutic control and associated reductions in serious adverse events associated with self-management would be exaggerated in comparison to UK models of care.

The PSM trial (SMART) was the largest UK-based RCT of self-management[3] and was not included in either of the previous reviews, as it was published later. There were 337 patients randomised to PSM intervention and 280 to routine care; in which 90/337

(24.5%) did not complete the training phase; and 193/337 (57%) of patients randomised completed the 12 months' allocated intervention. There was no significant difference in per cent time in range, (PSM 70% versus routine care 68%). These results agreed with those of other UK-based studies that control in UK routine care is good and, therefore, PSM is less likely to show any improvement.[4-5]

Cost-effectiveness data

The cost-effectiveness of PSM needs further investigation. One US study was identified that investigated cost.[6] The cost of home monitoring was approximately half that of routine care over an eight-week period, with costs based only on the cost of the monitor and test cartridges, compared with hospital laboratory tests. Other costs, such as transport for the patient and clinic overheads, were not included. The authors stated that if improved control reduced the risk of thromboembolic or haemorrhagic complications, the savings associated with home monitoring would be substantial.

One German study[7] demonstrated a 50% reduction in costs associated with self-management compared with routine care. Routine care, however, comprised patients being monitored by the physician office system and the analysis included instances of poor control and high rates of complications.

From the UK perspective, comparison with hospital clinic attendance and primary care-based management must be considered. One striking feature of all the papers reviewed is the high frequency of testing encouraged by the self-management model. Testing is recommended between every three and seven days, with increased frequency of testing should control deteriorate. This level of testing would be extremely costly and it is not clear why this frequency of testing is required. In comparison, stable patients in the clinic setting may only be tested at ten- to 13-week intervals.

The cost-effectiveness report from the SMART trial with two-weekly testing showed that overall mean healthcare costs for PSM were significantly higher than routine care.[8]

The principal findings from SMART were that around 25% of patients were willing and able to perform PSM; therapeutic control and adverse events were similar to routine care (70% time in range), while the costs from the NHS perspective were around £350, compared with around £100 for routine care.

The authors concluded that PSM did not appear to be cost-effective but may have other benefits, relieving pressure on traditional clinics.

In a survey sent to 538 anticoagulation clinic providers in the USA, barriers to self-testing were evaluated.[9] Three-quarters (75%) of respondents stated that some reimbursement for the cost of self-testing devices and supplies would increase the likelihood of clinics recommending self-testing. Another US study concluded that POC activity is resource intensive and, as healthcare budgets get tighter and staffing shortages grow, patient outcome must be weighed against available resources to determine optimum testing strategies.[10] Although this comment was not aimed specifically at self-management, it is obviously applicable to the UK healthcare budget as well.

Training for self-management

Currently, there are few formal training programmes for patients in the UK. However, data from the SMART trial suggest that a programme comprising two three-hour sessions – covering both practical and theoretical aspects, including quality assurance – is sufficient for the majority of patients.[11]

In Germany, around 90,000 patients currently manage their own anticoagulation therapy and there is a nationally approved, formalised training programme. As such, it is similar in concept to the National Asthma Training Centre (now Education for Health) in the UK, which provides training for healthcare professionals who then disseminate this training to patients.[12] The Association of Self-Management of Anticoagulation (Arbeitsgemeinschaft Selbstkontrolle der Antikoagulation e.V. [ASA]) has established a series of training centres across Germany. The association organises seminars to train the instructors (the doctors and nurses establishing home monitoring with their patients) and, in addition, to train patients.

For the trainers, the courses cover:
- Theoretical and pharmaceutical aspects of anticoagulation
- A training outline demonstrating the equipment to be used by the patients
- A practical session using the POCT systems.

The patient programme comprises:
- Theoretical aspects of anticoagulation management
- Indications for anticoagulation – how to monitor the blood
- Frequency of coagulation monitoring
- Problems with monitoring
- Interaction between anticoagulants and other medications
- Influences of nutrition, alcohol, intercurrent illness and travel
- Recording of test results
- Recognising and treating complications
- Overlapping heparin therapy
- Vaccinations
- Endocarditis prophylaxis.

The practical session includes:
- Operating the coagulation monitor
- Practising a coagulation test
- Practising an internal quality control test
- Correct finger stick procedure
- Possible sources of error
- Recording test results.

Quality assurance and frequency of testing

While quality control is deemed essential for hospital laboratories and primary care clinics undertaking INR measurements, the issue of both internal and external quality control for patients measuring their own INR has not previously been addressed.

One study evaluated four different methods of EQA in terms of effectiveness, compliance and patient satisfaction.[13] One group participated in a formal EQA scheme (UK National External Quality Assessment Service [UK NEQAS]) every three months using lyophilised samples sent to their home and the other group were asked to perform the same UK NEQAS test under the supervision of the research team three-monthly at their general practice.

Two other methods of external quality control were evaluated; first with INR results from venous samples sent to the local laboratory compared with contemporaneous POC capillary samples at the practice using the patient's POC system, and second, with INR results from the patient POC system capillary sample tests compared to results from a POC system weekly quality control, tested using samples from NEQAS at the practice, POC to POC.

The study demonstrated that patients were willing and able to perform EQA reliably, with a range of methods available to suit individual choice. Patients can utilise a formal scheme previously only used by healthcare professionals. As a result, there have been substantial developments in EQA activity for PSM; first, a follow-up study to evaluate PSM and EQA activity since the QAASM trial concluded showed that EQA was being was utilised by 80% of patients,[14] and second, UK NEQAS set up an EQA scheme specifically for patients (see Chapter 4).

Recommendations for the future

PST and PSM are becoming widespread and the systems are extensively advertised and easily available to purchase. Clinical supervision for PST and PSM is usually undertaken by the healthcare professional who has trained the patient to use the POC system. PST is particularly useful for those patients who are quite capable and enthusiastic to test their INR using a POC device but who are not confident to make dosage decisions; therefore, a healthcare professional would advise on dosing.

Currently clinicians, both in primary and secondary care, have expressed anxieties about patients' ability with both PST and PSM, particularly PSM, where dosing decisions are made by the patient. They have concerns over lack of guidelines and resources to cope with this additional model of care. It is clear that PST with PSM is clinically effective in patients' hands. It offers the patient an opportunity for a more flexible and convenient approach to one aspect of their healthcare and it is likely that there will be a demand now that test strips are on the Drug Tariff.

It is clear that standardisation of training and practical guidelines for PST and PSM are a pressing requirement and there has been some progression to address this subject.

Guidelines for clinical supervision of self-testing/management have been produced after consultation with some of the GPs, practice nurses and patients involved in the self-management trial, based on the recommendations for patient self-management produced on behalf of the British Society for Haematology Task Force for Haemostasis and Thrombosis.[15,16] The guidelines include advice on which patients to accept for self-testing or management of warfarin; quality control issues; frequency of testing; follow-up; dosing advice and equipment required.

Criteria for accepting patients to self-test/manage

● Patients on long-term warfarin only, using a POC device with an acceptable evaluation by an expert body such as the NHS Purchasing and Supply Agency, with a stated INR target in line with accepted guidelines and clinical practice.[15]
● Patients trained in self-testing and/or management of warfarin dosage to a standard acceptable to both the patient and the person with clinical responsibility.[15]
● An agreement signed by the patient and healthcare professional clinically responsible to undertake the measures listed below.

Follow-up

Follow-up review is agreed on an individual basis. Frequency of testing should be agreed by the responsible clinician. It is recommended that the patient is seen at least every six months.[15]

Documentation

INR results and dates, quality control results and any problems are documented accurately. (The yellow record book used widely by anticoagulant clinics can be used by the patient to record INR results and date of next test.)

Internal quality control

IQC, a simple test provided by the manufacturers, is performed and recorded at least every six months, or with every new box of test strips, or if an unusual result is obtained or after an unusual occurrence which may affect results (for example, dropping the machine).

External quality assessment

The use of an EQA programme (for example, the UK NEQAS for Blood Coagulation), is recommended.

There are two other methods of EQA, which may be more appropriate for some patients.

● The INR result from a venous sample taken at the follow-up clinic is sent to the local laboratory and compared with a simultaneous POC sample at the practice using the patient's POC system. The INR results should be within 0.5.
● The INR results from the patient's POC system can be compared to the result from a POC system used in the practice clinic, which is quality-controlled using samples from UK NEQAS, POC to POC. The INR results should be within 0.5.

Management of warfarin dosage

If a patient is self-managing their warfarin, an agreed algorithm for dosage of warfarin is followed and the clinician responsible contacted for advice if the patient decided to override the algorithm or if the INR result is greater than 5.0.

Advice and support and clinical responsibility

The INR test is performed at a specified weekday and time, agreed with the clinician responsible to enable easy access for advice if necessary. (All telephone contacts should be recorded within the patient notes.)

Disposal of waste and equipment

Patients dispose of needles safely in an appropriate container and other contaminated material wrapped up carefully and placed in the usual waste bin. Sharps boxes should be disposed of at point of purchase.

Responsibility is taken by the patient for ordering supplies of equipment directly from the manufacturer or on prescription if appropriate. Test strips and IQC materials are refrigerated at a temperature of 2–8°C (normal refrigerator temperature).

End of agreement

The clinician responsible is informed if the patient is intending to move away or to stop self-testing/management, so that arrangements can be made for an alternative method of management.

Summary

- Patient self-testing (PST) with patient self-management (PSM) has been found in a systematic review to be associated with a significant one-third reduction in major haemorrhage, and a non-significant reduction in the self-management group alone.
- The authors did state limitations to the review in that variability of care in control groups potentially affected the comparisons.
- PST and PSM are becoming widespread and the systems are extensively advertised and easily available to purchase.
- It is clear that standardisation of training and practical guidelines for PST and PSM are a pressing requirement and there has been some progression to address this subject.
- Guidelines for clinical supervision of PST/PSM have been produced after consultation based on the recommendations for PSM produced on behalf of the British Society for Haematology Task Force for Haemostasis and Thrombosis.
- One study demonstrated that patients were willing and able to perform EQA reliably, with a range of methods available to suit individual choice.

References

1. Heneghan C, Alonsa-Coello P, Garcia-Alamino JM *et al.* Self-monitorig of oral anticoagulation: a systematic review and meta-analysis. *Lancet* 2006; **367:** 404–411.
2. Fitzmaurice DA, Gardiner C, Kitchen S *et al.* An evidence-based review and guidelines for patient self-testing and management of oral anticoagulation *Br J Haematol* 2005; **131:**156–165.
3. Fitzmaurice DA, Murray ET, McCahon D *et al.* Self management of oral anticoagulation: a randomised trial. *BMJ* 2005; **331:** 1057.
4. Gardiner C, Williams K, Mackie IJ, Machin SJ, Cohen H. Patient self-testing is a reliable and acceptable alternative to laboratory INR monitoring. *Br J Haematol* 2005; **128:** 242–247.
5. Khan TI, Kamali F, Kesteven P, Avery P, Wynne H. The value of education and self monitoring in the management of warfarin therapy in older patients with unstable control of anticoagulation. *Br J Haematol* 2004; **126:** 557–564.
6. Anderson DR, Harrison L, Hirsh J. Evaluation of a portable prothrombin time monitor for home use by patients

who require long-term oral anticoagulant therapy. *Arch Intern Med* 1993; **153:** 1441–1447.

7. Bernado A. Experience with patient self-management of oral anticoagulation. *J Thromb Thrombolysis* 1995; **2:** 321–325.

8. Jowett S, Bryan S, Murray E *et al*. Patient self-management of anticoagulation therapy: a trial-based cost-effectiveness analysis. *Br J Haematol* 2006; **134:** 632–639.

9. Wittkowsky AK, Sekreta CM, Nutescu EA, Ansell J. Barriers to patient self-testing of prothrombin time: national survey of anticoagulation practitioners. *Pharmacotherapy* 2005; **25:** 265–269.

10. Nichols JH. Quality in point-of-care testing. *Expert Rev Mol Diagn* 2003; **3:** 563–572.

11. Fitzmaurice DA, Murray ET, Gee KM, Allan TF, Hobbs FD. A randomised controlled trial of patient self management of oral anticoagulation treatment compared with primary care management. *J Clin Pathol* 2002; **55:** 845–849.

12. Bisley C. A day in the life of an asthma nurse. *Asthma J* 1997; **2:** 152–154.

13. Murray ET, Jennings I, Kitchen D *et al*. Quality assurance for anticoagulation self management: QAASM a cluster randomised trial. *Journal of Thrombosis and Haemostasis* (Online Accepted Articles) doi:10.1111/j.1538-7836.2007.02875.

14. McCahon D, Murray ET, Jowett S *et al*. Patient self management of oral anticoagulation in routine care in the UK. *J Clin Pathol* 2007; **60:** 1263–1267.

15. Fitzmaurice DA, Machin SJ, BSH Task Force for Haemostasis and Thrombosis. Recommendations for patients undertaking self management of oral anticoagulation. *BMJ* 2001; **323:** 985–989.

16. Haemostasis and Thrombosis Task Force for the British Committee for Standards in Haematology. Guidelines on oral anticoagulation: third edition. *Br J Haematol* 1998; **101:** 374–387.

Chapter 11

The new oral anticoagulation era

Dr P Rose

Learning outcome

● **An understanding of new drugs to replace warfarin targeting different stages in the pro-coagulant pathway**

For more than 40 years, a new oral anticoagulant to replace warfarin has been the goal for many scientists, clinicians and patients alike. The ideal anticoagulant during this time period has been well defined; namely, to be effective orally, without significant interaction with other drugs, including alcohol, requiring no laboratory monitoring, readily reversible and without increased bleeding risk. Unfortunately, the last is incompatible with an effective anticoagulant. Many of the other requirements have, however, now been met by the new antithrombin and anti-Xa inhibitors. Figure 11.1 illustrates the large number of drugs currently under development targeting different stages in the pro-coagulant pathway. To date, these agents are continuing to undergo Phase II and III studies to assess the efficacy and safety issues, particularly surrounding the use of extended anticoagulant treatment. Table 11.1 (page 94) shows the properties of some of the more advanced anticoagulants.

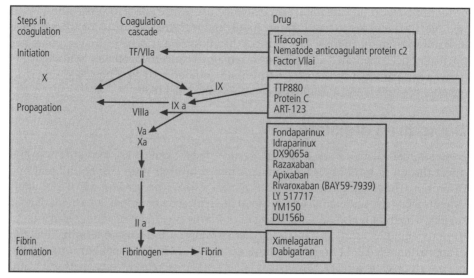

Figure 11.1. Drugs in development and their action on the pro-coagulant pathway

The first of the new order of oral anticoagulants to be licensed for orthopaedic thromboprophylaxis was ximelagatran. This drug shows good oral absorption and is bioconverted to its active form melagatran. The drug reaches a peak concentration at two hours, with low plasma protein binding of less than 15%. Drug clearance (80%) is by the renal system with a plasma half-life of four to five hours. Unlike warfarin, ximelagatran has a wide therapeutic window; thus, routine monitoring of laboratory coagulation tests is not required. The direct thrombin inhibitor inactivates free and fibrin bound thrombin. Furthermore, as it does not readily bind to plasma proteins, unlike heparin, a more predictable anticoagulant response is achieved. Unlike warfarin, it is unaffected by, and does not itself alter, the pharmacokinetics of other drugs metabolised via the cytochrome P450 pathway.

At the time of its launch, there was considerable reason for optimism, with ximelagatran meeting most of the criteria for an ideal oral anticoagulant. The initial licence indication was for the prevention of venous thromboembolism (VTE) in patients undergoing orthopaedic surgery. The METHRO and EXPRESS studies[1,2] showed a non-inferiority for ximelagatran compared with low molecular weight heparin (LMWH) for asymptomatic VTE post-orthopaedic surgery. Ximelagatran was given as a subcutaneous injection perioperatively, followed by the oral agent twice daily in the postoperative period. No difference in radiological or clinical endpoints were observed in terms of venous thromboembolic disease, with a non-significant increased bleeding with ximelagatran. Subsequent studies looking at the use of ximelagatran – both in the treatment of venous thromboembolic disease and, in the longer term, atrial fibrillation – were undertaken. In the THRIVE study,[3] the efficacy compared to LMWH was established in patients with symptomatic VTE, with or without pulmonary embolism. Unfortunately, abnormalities in the liver enzyme ALT began to emerge, with more than a threefold increase in this enzyme noted in around 9% of patients. Withdrawal of the drug routinely resulted in rapid resolution of the biochemical abnormality. In total, more than 20,000 patients received this agent; however, a very small number of patients began to be identified with hepatic failure on extended use. AstraZeneca took the unexpected step shortly thereafter to halt further studies and withdraw the drug for all its licence indications from the market. The cause of the idiosyncratic hepatic drug response has not to date been identified and, therefore, remains a concern for all new anticoagulants under trial, particularly the direct thrombin inhibitors. It has, however, served to enhance the surveillance of similar agents currently under trial.

Dabigatran etexilate

Dabigatran etexilate is a prodrug that is converted to dabigatran, a potent reversible direct thrombin inhibitor. Like ximelagatran, it inhibits both clot-bound and free thrombin. The drug is currently licensed for primary prevention of VTE in adult patients who have undergone elective total hip replacement or total knee replacement surgery. The drug is also under investigation for the treatment of venous and arterial thromboembolic disorders. The drug is active orally with the mean terminal half-life of approximately 12–14 hours in volunteers and 14–17 hours in patients undergoing major orthopaedic surgery. The drug is largely (85%) excreted by renal pathways, and patients with moderate renal impairment or elderly patients require a dose reduction

Table 11.1. Properties of anticoagulant drugs

	Argatroban	Hirudin	Bivalirudin	Ximelagatran
Type of action	Bivalent DTI	Bivalent DTI	Active site DTI	Active site DTI
Administration	IV	IV	IV	Oral
Half-life	45 mins	80 mins	25 mins	4 hrs
Clearance	Hepatic	Renal	Proteolysis	Renal
Reversible	Yes	Slow	Rapid	Yes

DTI = direct thrombin inhibito. IV = intravenous. SC = subcutaneous

to 75 mg for the first dose postoperatively, followed by 150 mg per day. It currently meets many of the criteria for an ideal anticoagulant; in particular. it has a low level of drug interactions. The cytochrome P450 pathway is not involved in the formation or metabolism of dabigatran. The drug has a fast onset and offset of action and is not affected by interactions with food. Due to its wide therapeutic window, the drug does not require laboratory monitoring of coagulation tests.

Orthopaedic thromboprophylaxis

Dabigatran etexilate has been has been trialled in over 8,000 patients undergoing orthopaedic surgery. The Phase III trial programme comprised three double-blind, double-dummy, randomised studies comparing the use of dabigatran etexilate to enoxaparin. In the RE-MODEL and RE-NOVATE studies[4,5] the first dose of dabigatran etexilate was given one to four hours post-surgery, compared with enoxaparin 40 mg subcutaneously given the evening before surgery. The length of treatment was six to ten days post total knee replacement and 28–35 days post total hip replacement. In a third study, RE-MOBILIZE,[6] treatment post total knee replacement was for 12–15 days post-surgery with a first dose of dabigatran after six to 12 hours, with enoxaparin given 12–24 hours post-surgery at 30 mg twice daily. The major exclusion criteria included patients with bleeding diathesis, a history of recent bleeding events including haemorrhagic strokes, severe liver disease, abnormal liver function, severe renal insufficiency, non-steroidal anti-inflammatory drug therapy, or active malignancy.

Dabigatran was demonstrated to show non-inferiority versus enoxaparin 40 mg per day for the prevention of VTE post hip[5] and post knee[4] surgery. It was, however, found to be inferior versus enoxaparin 30 mg twice daily in the prevention of VTE post total knee replacement.[6] The agent demonstrated a similar safety profile to enoxaparin in all three studies. The recommendation from all three studies is for dabigatran to be given as a single capsule 110 mg one to four hours post-surgery. Thereafter, two capsules

Fondaparinux	Idraparinux	Dabigatran	Rivaroxaban
Indirect Xa inhibitor	Indirect Xa inhibitor	DTI	Direct Xa inhibitor
IV/SC	SC	Oral	Oral
15 hrs	130 hrs	12-14 hrs	5.2-9.2 hrs
Renal	Renal	Renal	Renal 66%, faecal/ biliary 28%
No	No	No	No

(220 mg) once daily for ten days post knee surgery and for 28–35 days after elective hip replacement surgery.

This agent, therefore, meets most of the requirements for an ideal oral anticoagulant agent and has the potential to greatly simplify anticoagulant thromboprophylaxis post-orthopaedic surgery. No single method for rapid reversal of anticoagulant activity is available for this agent.

Rivaroxaban

Rivaroxaban is an oral, direct, and highly selective inhibitor of activated factor X. In the Phase III trial programme for the prevention of VTE after orthopaedic surgery from the RECORD studies,[7] it has been shown to be superior in the efficacy for the composite endpoint of deep vein thrombosis (DVT), non-fatal pulmonary embolism (PE) and all-cause mortality when compared with enoxaparin when given at 40 mg subcutaneously once per day or 30 mg subcutaneously twice per day. Rivaroxaban has a high oral bioavailability, with a peak plasma concentration two to four hours after oral administration. It is primarily excreted by the renal (66%) and faecal/biliary routes (28%). The half-life in the elderly extends (from 5.7–9.0 hours in patients aged 22–45 years) to 11–13 hours, mainly due to reduced renal clearance. Drug interactions are much less commonly seen than with warfarin, although agents that are strong inducers or inhibitors of cytochrome P3A4 and plasma glycoprotein, such as ketoconazole and rifampicin, may modify anticoagulant effect. Overall, however, the safety profile is promising, with low bleeding incidence similar to that of enoxaparin.

Conclusion

It does finally appear that a new era of oral anticoagulant management has arrived. There will, however, remain concerns about the longer-term safety of these agents, given the previous experience with ximelagatran. The potential for these agents to alter the delivery of anticoagulant services with no laboratory monitoring and less concern about serious drug interaction should make extended thromboprophylaxis and extended treatment more readily achievable. The rate of change and uptake of the new agents is, however, impossible to predict. Overall, the change in management of oral anticoagulation from secondary to primary care will be facilitated as these agents gain wider licence for thromboprophylaxis and treatment. These agents may also have an impact on quality of life for patients, particularly those who have problems attending anticoagulation clinics on a regular basis.

Summary

- The ideal anticoagulant needs to be effective orally, without significant interaction with other drugs, including alcohol, requiring no laboratory monitoring, readily reversible and without increased bleeding risk.
- There is a large number of drugs currently under development targeting different stages in the pro-coagulant pathway.
- The potential for these agents to alter the delivery of anticoagulant services with no laboratory monitoring and less concern about serious drug interaction should make extended thromboprophylaxis and extended treatment more readily achievable.
- The change in management of oral anticoagulation from secondary to primary care will be facilitated as these agents gain wider licence for thromboprophylaxis and treatment.

References

1. Eriksson BI, Bergqvist D, Kälebo P *et al*. Ximelagatran and melagatran compared with dalteparin for prevention of venous thromboembolism after total hip or knee replacement: the METHRO II randomised trial. *Lancet* 2002; **360:** 1441–1447.
2. Eriksson BI, Agnelli G, Cohen AT *et al*. The direct thrombin inhibitor malagatran followed by oral ximelagatran compared with enoxaparin for the prevention of venous thromboembolism after total hip or knee replacement: the EXPRESS study. *J Thromb Haemost* 2003; **1:** 2490–2496.
3. Shulman S, Wåhlander K, Lundström T *et al*. Secondary prevention of venous thromboembolism with the oral direct thrombin inhibitor Ximelagatran. *N Eng J Med* 2003; **349:** 1713–1721.
4. Eriksson BI, Dahl OE, Rosencher N *et al*. Oral dabigatran etexilate vs subcutaneous enoxaparin for the prevention of venous thromboembolism after total knee replacement: the RE-MODEL randomized trial. *J Thromb Haemost* 2007; **5:** 2178–2185.
5. Eriksson BI, Dahl OE, Rosencher N *et al*. Dabigatran etexilate versus enoxaparin for prevention of venous thromboembolism after total hip replacement: a randomised, double-blind, non-inferiority trial. *Lancet* 2007; **370:** 949–956.
6. Friedman RJ, Caprini JA, Comp PC *et al*. Dabigatran Etexilate vs. Enoxaparin in preventing venous thromboembolism following total knee arthroplasty. *J Thromb Haemost* 2007; **5**(Suppl 2): O-W-051.
7. Eriksson BI, Borris LC, Friedman RJ *et al*. Rivaroxaban versus enoxaparin for thromboprophylaxis after hip arthroplasty. *N Engl J Med* 2008; **358:** 2765–2775.

Chapter 12

Prevention and treatment of venous thromboembolism

Dr L Roberts

Dr R Arya

Learning outcomes

- **Risk assessment for venous thromboembolism will enable delivery of appropriate thromboprophylaxis**
- **The use of integrated diagnostic and treatment strategies for deep vein thrombosis (DVT) allows safe and effective outpatient management of most patients**

Prevention of venous thromboembolism

Venous thromboembolism (VTE), comprising deep vein thrombosis (DVT) and pulmonary embolism (PE), is a major public health problem. VTE affects 100 per 100,000 population per year and in England alone causes thousands of deaths annually. Large population-based studies have shown that factors associated with hospitalisation account for half the attributable risk of VTE. In 2005, the House of Commons Health Committee report highlighted the urgent need to prevent avoidable deaths from VTE. Two years later, two significant pieces of national guidance were published: the Chief Medical Officer's independent VTE expert working group's report, which recommended an integrated approach to VTE prevention (Table 12.1, page 98) and the National Institute for Health and Clinical Excellence (NICE) guidance regarding VTE risk reduction in surgical patients. These initiatives provide an impetus for implementation of thrombosis prevention across the spectrum of healthcare, from acute trusts into the community.

VTE risk assessment and thromboprophylaxis

The evidence that appropriate thromboprophylaxis reduces the burden of VTE is well established and detailed in the American College of Chest Physicians (ACCP) clinical practice guidelines (2008) on prevention of VTE. To prevent VTE, the at-risk patient has to be identified, counselled, then given appropriate prophylaxis. Risk assessment triggers the thromboprophylaxis pathway, hence the recommendation that every hospitalised patient be risk assessed on admission. There are generally two approaches to risk assessment. The first is an individualised or 'opt-in' approach, wherein the risk of VTE

Table 12.1. Summary of independent VTE expert working group's recommendations

- Systematic and integrated approach to VTE prevention
- Documented risk assessment of every patient on admission to hospital
- VTE risk assessment is incorporated in trust risk management frameworks with core standards set by the Department of Health
- Improvement of public and professional education with regard to VTE
- Implementation of strategies for thromboprophylaxis
- Establishment of exemplar centres to promote best practice

in each patient is considered, based on his or her predisposing factors and current illness or procedure. The second is the exclusion or 'opt-out' approach, which delivers group-specific prophylaxis routinely for all patients in the major target groups. In future, the process of VTE risk assessment might extend into the community; for instance, patients may be risk-assessed in primary care before hospitalisation for high-risk elective procedures. In medical patients, the ongoing VTE risk might need to be considered in nursing home residents and other patients following discharge after treatment for an acute illness.

The patient at risk for VTE should receive appropriate thromboprophylaxis, which might include pharmacological and mechanical measures. Injections of low molecular weight heparin (LMWH) are currently the mainstay of pharmacological prophylaxis in high-risk medical and surgical patients for reasons of efficacy, safety and convenience. Of note, aspirin, due to its limited efficacy, is unsuitable for prophylaxis of VTE. For some surgical and medical patients, the increased risk of VTE continues beyond the period of hospitalisation and extended prophylaxis may be warranted. The use of LMWH for extended prophylaxis in the community raises resource issues for primary care around arrangements for administration of injections, blood tests to exclude heparin-induced thrombocytopenia and funding for the drugs. In the future, oral agents such as the direct thrombin inhibitors and anti-factor Xa inhibitors are likely to provide safe and effective thromboprophylaxis and would facilitate delivery of extended prophylaxis regimens.

VTE diagnosis

VTE may be difficult to diagnose clinically and, furthermore, many cases may be silent. Approximately one-quarter of those presenting with suspected diagnosis of VTE are confirmed to have an event. For those presenting with symptoms typical of VTE, such as painful swollen leg or dyspnoea and pleuritic chest pain, integrated diagnostic strategies have improved diagnostic accuracy and ensured patient safety and are cost-effective. Such strategies rely on a combination of clinical pre-test probability, D-dimers and appropriate imaging (Figure 12.1, page 99). When VTE is suspected, assessment of the

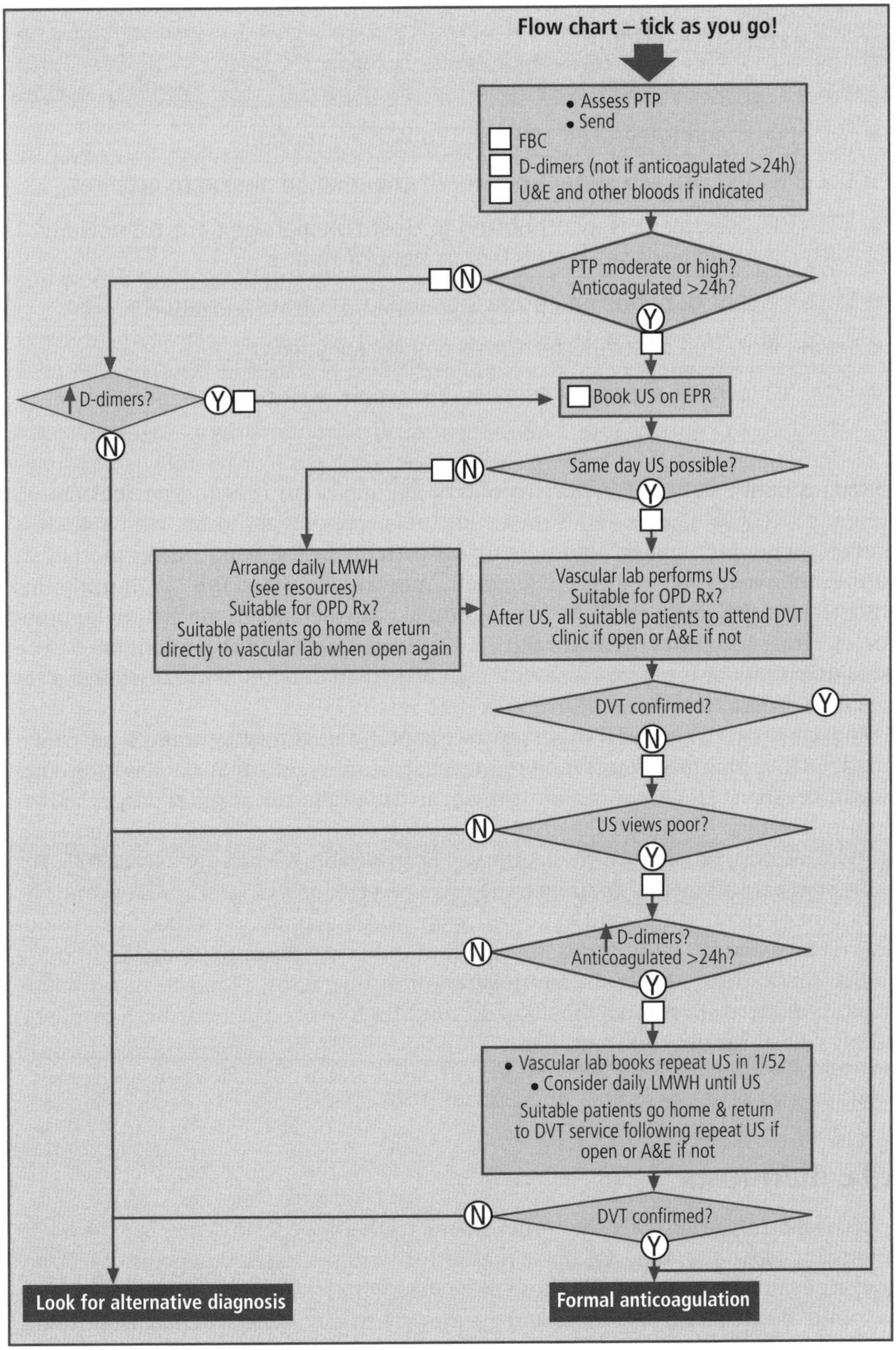

Figure 12.1. Flow chart demonstrating investigation of possible deep vein thrombosis (DVT).
EPR = electronic patient record. FBC = full blood count. LMWH = low molecular weight heparin. OPD Rx = outpatient
department prescription. PTP = pre-test probability. U&E = Urea & electrolytes. US = ultrasonography

Courtesy of King's Thrombosis Centre, King's College Hospital.

pre-test probability (PTP) is the first step. Wells and colleagues developed a clinical prediction rule for DVT based on symptoms, risk factors and signs to risk stratify patients into low-, moderate- and high-risk groups (Table 12.2), with DVT subsequently detected in 3%, 17% and 75% of patients respectively. D-dimers, the smallest breakdown product of a fibrin clot, are useful in combination with a low PTP in ruling out DVT. For instance, Kearon and colleagues (2001) found the combination of a negative D-dimer and low PTP to have a high negative predictive value for DVT, at 99.4%. In a randomised study, Wells and colleagues (2003) found that just 0.4% of patients with a low PTP and negative D-dimer had confirmed VTE during three-month follow-up. Thus, DVT can be excluded in such patients without further investigation.

Venography, the gold standard imaging test for DVT diagnosis, is invasive, expensive and cumbersome and has almost completely been replaced by compression ultrasonography as the initial imaging test: DVT is diagnosed by the inability to compress the thrombosed vein (Figure 12.2, page 101). Ultrasonography is highly sensitive (97–100%) and specific (98–99%) for proximal DVT but less accurate generally for distal (calf vein) DVT, with sensitivity of 70% and specificity of 60%. The rate of symptomatic VTE was reported by Stevens and colleagues (2004) to be less than 1% in patients who had anticoagulation withheld after a single negative ultrasound of the lower limb venous system. The British Committee for Standards in Haematology (BCSH) (2004) suggests those with a negative D-dimer require no further imaging and those with a positive D-dimer should have anticoagulation withheld and repeat ultrasonography at one week to enable detection of a DVT extending into the proximal vasculature. There is debate whether it is desirable to detect distal DVT, as it is rarely complicated by PE, but most expert opinion would favour diagnosis and treatment of distal DVT, as this provides symptomatic relief, reduces proximal extension and prevents recurrence. In some quarters there is an interest in community DVT clinics, in

Table 12.2. Wells's pre-test probability score for DVT

	Points
Active malignancy (on treatment/completed within 6 months/palliation)	1
Paralysis, plaster	1
Bed-bound for more than 3 days, surgery within 4 weeks	1
Tenderness along the venous system	1
Swelling of the entire leg	1
Calf swollen more than 3cm	1
Pitting oedema	1
Collateral veins	1
Alternative diagnosis more likely	-2

0 = low, 1-2 = moderate, ≥3 = high risk

Images courtesy of Dr David Goss, Vascular Scientist, King's College Hospital, London.

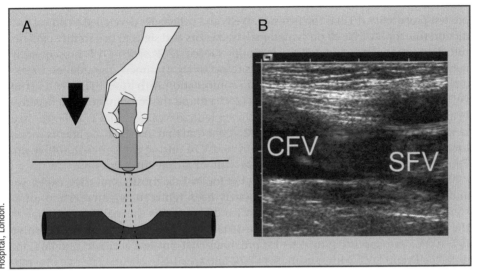

Figure 12.2. A: Compression ultrasound demonstrating direct venous compression with the transducer. B: Superficial femoral vein (SFV) occluded with thrombus extending into common femoral vein (CFV)

parallel with the move towards community anticoagulation. PTP assessment and point-of-care D-dimer testing are easily undertaken in primary care but ultrasound examination is usually performed in secondary care; impedance or strain-gauge plethysmography, often recommended for community use, is insufficiently sensitive or specific for use as a stand-alone test for DVT. Lastly, diagnosis of PE has, like DVT, been improved by use of diagnostic algorithms employing clinical PTP, D-dimer and suitable imaging as described in the British Thoracic Society guidelines (2003). Computerised tomography pulmonary angiography (CTPA) is the imaging modality of choice, being highly sensitive to a subsegmental level and also revealing alternative diagnoses such as cancer or infection.

When VTE is diagnosed, the setting in which the event has occurred must also be considered. Common risk factors include recent hospitalisation for surgery or with an acute medical illness, pregnancy, hormonal risk factors, cancer and thrombophilia (most commonly factor V Leiden). Cancer accounts for up to 20% of VTE events: VTE might be the presenting symptom, or arise during the course of malignant disease. Routine screening for occult malignancy at presentation remains controversial, as evidence that this translates into an improved clinical outcome is lacking. Unless there are clinical indicators of malignancy, a thorough clinical assessment, routine laboratory tests and chest radiography should suffice.

VTE treatment

Anticoagulation is the mainstay of therapy for VTE, aiming to relieve symptoms, prevent further thrombus extension and embolisation and, in the long term, prevent recurrence. Thrombolysis or surgical thrombectomy/embolectomy is restricted to selected patients with haemodynamic instability due to massive PE or critical limb ischaemia secondary to DVT as described in the ACCP guidelines (2008). Anticoagulation should be initiated on confirmation of the diagnosis of VTE. In situations where there is a delay in diagnosis, patients with suspected VTE should be empirically anticoagulated while awaiting diagnostic imaging. Baseline bloods for platelet count, coagulation and liver and renal function should be taken before initiation of anticoagulation.

LMWH is the preferred agent for initiation of anticoagulation due to ease of administration with once-daily subcutaneous injection, the lack of need for monitoring and the lower risk of heparin-induced thrombocytopenia. Additionally, a Cochrane review undertaken by van Dongen in 2004 found fewer deaths, and less major haemorrhage and recurrent VTE, with LMWH compared with unfractionated heparin (UFH). Warfarin should be commenced once the diagnosis has been confirmed, unless contraindicated, with a target international normalised ratio (INR) of 2.5 recommended by the BCSH and ACCP guidelines. LMWH should be continued for at least five days and until the INR has been therapeutic for 24 hours. The initial rise in INR with warfarin commencement is due to decreased factor VII levels, but full anticoagulation is not achieved until the remaining vitamin K-dependent factors (II, IX, X) fall, which takes three to five days.

Most patients with a diagnosis of DVT can be safely managed on an outpatient basis. This may be inappropriate in patients with significant comorbid illness, pregnancy or those unlikely to comply with therapy. Possible models of ambulant care range from regular attendance at the hospital DVT clinic to domiciliary care administered by outreach haemostasis nurses or by district nurses and GPs. Adequate analgesia should be provided and initial anticoagulation should be closely supervised to allow timely cessation of LMWH. Patients should be advised regarding symptoms that require further medical attention; namely, progressive breathlessness, new onset chest pain or pre-syncopal episodes, in addition to bleeding, and who to contact in such an event. It may be more appropriate to continue anticoagulation with LMWH alone in pregnancy, in patients with active malignancy and in intravenous drug users. Conversely, most patients diagnosed with PE are managed initially as an inpatient due to increased early morbidity and mortality. There is emerging evidence to support outpatient management for carefully selected patients at low risk of early complications, although this is far from universally practised.

The recommended duration of anticoagulation is determined by the site of thrombosis, in addition to the presence of precipitating risk factors. There are several studies examining VTE recurrence rates and duration of anticoagulation, summarised in the BCSH (2005) and ACCP guidance (2008); generally, longer periods of anticoagulation are superior to shorter periods for reducing VTE recurrence. At least six weeks of anticoagulation is recommended after calf vein thrombosis and at least three months after proximal DVT or PE. For patients with idiopathic VTE or permanent risk factors, at least six months of anticoagulation is recommended, with duration of anticoagulation reviewed case by case. Patients with recurrent unprovoked VTE should receive long-term anticoagulation. The latest ACCP guidance also recommends long-term treatment for patients with single unprovoked proximal DVT or PE in whom risk factors for bleeding are absent and good anticoagulation monitoring is achievable; this is not currently standard practice in the UK. Most experts consider the patient's clinical history to be the most important determinant of the length of anticoagulation, though laboratory studies may also provide useful information. In patients who receive long-term anticoagulation, the risk–benefit ratio for continuing treatment should be periodically reviewed.

VTE aftercare

Long-term complications of VTE include recurrent VTE, post-thrombotic syndrome (PTS) following DVT, and pulmonary hypertension following PE. Once anticoagulation has been discontinued, the risk of recurrence in patients with a first episode of VTE associated with a major transient risk factor is approximately 3% per year. In those with idiopathic VTE, or with a continuing risk factor, recurrence risk is 10% per year, with the greatest risk shortly after stopping treatment. PTS arises from damage to the deep venous system leading to a constellation of symptoms including pain, swelling, varicose eczema and venous ulceration. Kahn and Ginsberg reviewed the relationship between DVT and PTS in 2004 and describe its prevalence in up to 50% of patients post-DVT; severe PTS affects one in ten DVT patients. In 1997, Brandjes and colleagues demonstrated that correctly fitted grade II graduated elastic compression stockings (ECSs) effectively reduce the incidence of PTS. Patients should be fitted with these once the initial swelling has resolved following an acute DVT, with advice to continue wearing them for at least two years. Pulmonary hypertension is a rare complication of PE and will not be further discussed here.

Patient education is integral to the management of VTE: to ensure compliance with anticoagulation and attendance for INR monitoring, to facilitate compliance with ECSs post-DVT and for risk avoidance after completion of anticoagulation. All patients should be informed of situations predisposing to VTE, such as major abdominal/pelvic surgery, orthopaedic surgery, oral contraceptive pill/hormone replacement therapy, pregnancy and long-haul air travel. All patients should be counselled regarding future risk and appropriate thromboprophylaxis on completion of anticoagulation. With regard to long-haul travel, in most individuals common-sense measures should suffice, such as avoiding constrictive clothing and remaining mobile and well hydrated. In the presence of additional risk factors such as previous VTE, cancer or thrombophilia, additional prophylactic measures may be employed, such as anti-embolism stockings or single LMWH injections (at the prophylactic dose) given prior to each flight. The ACCP guidance (2008) specifically recommends against the use of aspirin for VTE prevention in this or any other setting.

The role of thrombophilia testing following completion of anticoagulation remains controversial. Thrombophilia studies are usually undertaken at least four weeks after discontinuation of warfarin. The results, 'positive' in 30–40% of Northern European patients and in less than 10% of black patients, might yield an insight into the reasons for occurrence of VTE in an individual and enable family studies, but are unlikely, in most cases, to affect treatment choice. The exception to this is strongly 'thrombophilic' individuals, who should be considered for long-term anticoagulation to reduce recurrent VTE; this might include those with antiphospholipid syndrome, inherited anticoagulant (antithrombin, protein C, protein S) deficiency and those with more than one allelic abnormality (such as homozygous factor V Leiden, heterozygosity for both factor V Leiden and prothrombin G20210A mutation). In addition to 'standard' thrombophilia testing, there is growing interest in the role for biomarkers in the risk stratification of patients following a first VTE: shortened activated partial thromboplastin time, elevated D-dimers and increased thrombin generation have been individually linked to VTE recurrence.

Summary

- Prevention of VTE entails documented risk assessment of all hospitalised patients and delivery of appropriate thromboprophylaxis.
- Integrated diagnostic strategies, comprising pre-test probability, D-dimer and appropriate imaging, may be used to diagnose VTE.
- Most DVT patients can be safely, effectively and conveniently treated as outpatients.
- Anticoagulation is the mainstay of treatment for VTE and comprises once-daily LMWH injections at the outset and vitamin K antagonists.
- For treatment of VTE with vitamin K antagonists, the target INR is 2.5 and duration of therapy is three to six months for most patients.
- In VTE associated with pregnancy, cancer and intravenous drug use, patients should be treated with LMWH injections alone.
- The aftercare of patients with VTE might include thrombophilia testing, advice regarding risk factors for VTE/suitable thromboprophylaxis in high-risk situations and management of complications such as PTS.

Further reading
House of Commons Health Committee. *The Prevention of Venous Thromboembolism in Hospitalised Patients.* London: The Stationery Office, 2005.
Department of Health. *Report of the independent expert working group on the prevention of venous thromboembolism in hospitalised patients.* London: DH, 2007.
National Institute for Health and Clinical Excellence. *Venous thromboembolism: reducing the risk of venous thromboembolism in inpatients undergoing surgery.* London: National Collaborating Centre for Acute Care, 2007.
Geerts WH, Bergqvist D, Pineo GF *et al.* Prevention of venous thromboembolism: American College of Chest Physicians Evidence-Based Clinical Practice Guidelines (8th Edition). *Chest* 2008; **133**(Suppl 6): S381–S453.
Wells PS. Integrated strategies for the diagnosis of venous thromboembolism. *J Thromb Haemost* 2007; **5**(Suppl 1): 41–50.
Wells PS, Anderson DR, Bormanis J *et al.* Value of assessment of pretest probability of deep-vein thrombosis in clinical management. *Lancet* 1997; **350:** 1795–1798.
Kearon C, Ginsberg JS, Douketis J *et al.* Management of suspected deep venous thromboembolism in outpatients by using clinical assessment and D-dimer testing. *Ann Intern Med* 2001; **135:** 108–111.
Wells PS, Anderson DR, Rodger M *et al.* Evaluation of D-dimer in the diagnosis of suspected deep-vein thrombosis. *N Engl J Med* 2003; **349:** 1227–1235.
Kyrle PA, Eichenger S. Deep vein thrombosis. *Lancet* 2005; **365:** 1163–1174.
Stevens SM, Elliott CG, Chan KJ, Egger MJ, Ahmed KM. Withholding anticoagulation after a negative result on duplex ultrasonography for suspected symptomatic deep venous thrombosis. *Ann Intern Med* 2004; **140:** 985–991.
Keeling DM, Mackie IJ, Moody A, Watson HG, The Haemostasis and Thrombosis Task Force of the British Committee for Standards in Haematology. The diagnosis of deep vein thrombosis in symptomatic outpatients and the potential for clinical assessment and D-dimer assays to reduce the need for diagnostic imaging. *Br J Haem.* 2004; **124:** 15–25.
British Thoracic Society Standards of Care Committee Pulmonary Embolism Guideline Development Group. British Thoracic Society guidelines for the management of suspected acute pulmonary embolism. *Thorax* 2003; **58:** 470–483.
Kearon C, Kahn SR, Agnelli G *et al.* Antithrombotic therapy for venous thromboembolic disease: American College of Chest Physicians Evidence-Based Clinical Practice Guidelines (8th Edition). *Chest* 2008; **133**(Suppl 6): S454–S545.
Van Dongen CJ, van der Belt AG, Prins MH, Lensing AW. Fixed dose subcutaneous low molecular weight heparins versus adjusted dose unfractionated heparin. *Cochrane Database Syst Rev* 2004; **4:** CD001100.

Baglin TP, Keeling DM, Watson HG, British Committee for Standards in Haematology. Guidelines on oral anticoagulation (warfarin): third edition – 2005 update. *Br J Haematol* 2006; **132:** 277–285.

Kahn SR, Ginsberg JS. Relationship between deep venous thrombosis and the postthrombotic syndrome. *Arch Int Med* 2004; **164:** 17–26.

Brandjes DP, Büller HR, Heijboer H *et al*. Randomised trial of effect of compression stockings in patients with symptomatic proximal-vein thrombosis. *Lancet* 1997; **349:** 759–762.

Index

108

Authors' contact details

Dr R Arya
Consultant Haematologist,
King's College Hospital,
Denmark Hill,
London
SE5 9RS.

Professor DA Fitzmaurice
Professor of Primary Care
Research,
Department of Primary Care
and General Practice,
University of Birmingham,
Edgbaston,
Birmingham
B15 2TT

Mr C Gardiner
Chief Biomedical Scientist,
Department of Haematology
Evaluation,
5th Floor North,
60 Whitfield Street,
London
W1T 4EU.

Dr S Jowett
Research Fellow,
Health Economics Facility,
School of Health and
Population Sciences,
Public Health Building,
University of Birmingham,
Edgbaston,
Birmingham
B15 2TT.

Dr P Kesteven
Consultant Haematologist,
Freeman Hospital,
Freeman Road, High Heaton,
Newcastle-upon-Tyne
NE7 7DN.

Mrs DP Kitchen
Point-of-care Co-ordinator,
UK NEQAS for Blood
Coagulation,
Rutledge Mews,
3 Southbourne Road,
Sheffield
S10 2QN.

Dr S Kitchen
Scientific Director,
UK NEQAS for Blood
Coagulation,
Rutledge Mews,
3 Southbourne Road,
Sheffield
S10 2QN.

Dr WA Lester
Consultant in Haematology,
Queen Elizabeth Hospital,
Edgbaston,
Birmingham
B15 2TH.

Professor SJ Machin
Consultant Haematologist,
Department of Haematology,
University College Hospitals,
250 Euston Road,
London
NW1 2PQ.

Dr ET Murray
Senior Lecturer,
Department of Primary Care
and General Practice,
University of Birmingham,
Edgbaston,
Birmingham
B15 2TT.

Dr JA Murray
Consultant Haematologist,
Queen Elizabeth Hospital,
Edgbaston,
Birmingham
B15 2TH.

Professor J Raftery
Wessex Institute for Health
Research and Development,
Mailpoint 728,
Boldrewood,
University of Southampton,
Southampton
SO16 7PX.

Dr L Roberts
Haematology Specialist
Registrar,
King's College Hospital,
Denmark Hill,
London
SE5 9RS.

Dr P Rose
Consultant Haematologist,
Warwick Hospital,
Lakin Road,
Warwick
CV34 5BW.

Professor ID Walker
Director,
UK NEQAS for Blood
Coagulation,
Rutledge Mews,
3 Southbourne Road,
Sheffield
S10 2QN.